The Compleat Herbal

Being a description of the origins, the lore, the characteristics, the types, and the prescribed uses of medicinal herbs, *including an alphabetical guide to all common medicinal plants.*

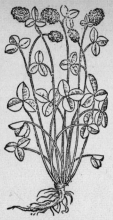 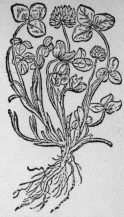

*Of CLOVERS there are many kinds wild in Britain. Some are very small, and, though abundant, are easily overlooked. The best known are the cultivated species figured on this page—the White, the Red, and the Purple. What plant TREFOIL OF AMERICA is one cannot suggest. TREACLE CLOVER was used as an antidote or counter-poison. A treacle was "a physical composition made of vipers and other ingredients" to the number of sixty! It was good for curing envenomed wounds, though if applied to wounds which were not envenomed it increased the pain by drawing to the wound "from far" those "humors" it must needs act against. The "Treacle Bible" has its name from its reading—"for there is no more Tryacle at Galaad."
—Jer. viii. 22.

HARE'S-FOOT TREFOIL has its furry flower-heads whitish with the long feathery points of its calyxes. The corollas are too small to greatly influence the colour.

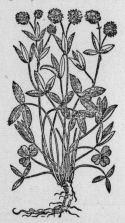 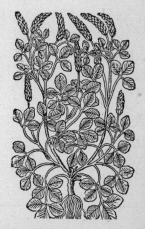

*Originally published in The Craftsmen's Plant-Book (1909).

The Compleat Herbal

Being a description of the origins, the lore, the characteristics, the types, and the prescribed uses of medicinal herbs, *including an alphabetical guide to all common medicinal plants.*

by Ben Charles Harris

Larchmont Books
Atlanta, Georgia

Notice: This book is meant as an informational guide for the prevention of disease. For conditions of ill-health, we recommend that you see a physician, pyschiatrist or other professional licensed to treat disease. These days, many medical practitioners are discovering that a strong nutritional program supports and fortifies whatever therapy they may use, as well as effectively preventing a recurrence of the illness.

Fourth Printing: *January, 1984*
Third Printing: *February, 1980*
Second Printing: *May, 1978*
First Printing: *April, 1975*

THE COMPLEAT HERBAL

Copyright © 1972 by Ben Charles Harris

Published by arrangement with Barre Publishers.
Library of Congress Catalog Card Number 77-185615.
Designed by Dwight Edward Agner.

ISBN 0-915962-15-2

Printed in the United States of America.

LARCHMONT BOOKS
*6255 Barfield Rd.
Atlanta, Ga. 30328*

Contents

Acknowledgments

I am beholden first of all to the original researchers listed in the bibliography, for their investigations into the historical backgrounds of herbal lore and into the diverse accomplishments of those "old makers of medicine" of past ages who have contributed so greatly to modern healing arts.

I am grateful also to Mr. Lewis Hodgkinson of the Worcester County Extension Service for reviewing the portion of the manuscript dealing with herbal lore and therapeutic treatments; to two of my informants of Indian ancestry, who wish to remain anonymous, for valuable advice and information and for their relating to me many of their childhood experiences; to Princess White Flower of the nearby Hassanamisco tribe, in Grafton, Mass., with sincere thanks for her constructive criticism of the chapter on the Indians; and especially to my devoted wife, Faye, whose patience and perseverance made this work all the more possible.

I am deeply indebted to the librarians of Worcester State College, Clark University, Holy Cross College, Assumption College, and Massachusetts College of Pharmacy, for their help and guidance in seeking out the needed sources of information.

Finally, I must acknowledge the assistance given to me on innumerable almost daily occasions by the indefatigable and most patient staff of the Telephone Information Service of the Worcester Public Library.

Ben Charles Harris

The Compleat Herbal

Introduction

This book germinated in the mid-1940s when a series of my
articles entitled "Superstitions and the Folklore of Herbs"
appeared in *Nature Outlook,* the publication of the Worcester
Museum of Natural History, after I gave a series of radio
talks under the same title. The research developed and ex-
panded over the next twenty-five years, as I lectured to inter-
ested groups as the museum's Curator of Economic Botany.

The history of herbal medicine is of course as old as man
himself, and our present knowledge is a product of thousands
of years of observation and trial and error by primitive peoples
all over the world, and codification and experimentation by the
great herbalists of the past 500 years. Modern medicine is but
a miniscule part of man's attempts to overcome disease; for
a million years before the hospital and the laboratory, man
searched for green medicine in the plants that grew all around
him. Thousands were remarkably effective, and after their uses
were established many plants took their common names from
the organ they benefited.

The legacy from the past, then, is an enormous one; and in
this book I pay tribute to the first herbalists of North America,
the Indians. They provided the early settlers with a spectrum
of herbal remedies which have been handed on down to this
very day. A method of identifying helpful herbs also developed

many centuries ago. Called the doctrine of signatures, it associates the remedy with outstanding characteristics—shape, color, and so on—of the plant. It is a fascinating approach, not only because of the satisfying symmetry of such correspondence, but because generally it is an accurate guide. I adopted the doctrine of signatures as a teaching aid in identifying medicinal herbs, and shall do so in this book.

Since the book is about herbal medicine—that is, herbs that heal—the notion of health, or, more precisely, lack of health, should be clear. What do we mean when we speak of disease, and then of its cure? The word *health* is derived from a Germanic root meaning "whole" or "wholesome." Health is a positive force, and disease, I feel, is the absence of health. Most illnesses are self-inflicted, either by ignorance or by intentional disregard of the few basic rules of healthy living. Foremost among the practices that encourage disease are faulty eating habits, intemperance, and the effects of stress—in short, general neglect of those fundamentals which promote health.

Modern man is ever seeking cures without examining the causes of disease. Certainly, in this enlightened age, one does not acquire dental caries because of unfluoridated drinking water, nor diabetes because of lack of insulin injections in childhood, nor various infectious disorders because of a lack of immunization. Feverish colds and bronchial disturbances are not caused by the lack of antibiotics. The warning signals—symptoms of disease—are often temporary if their causes are quickly eliminated and healthful practices follow. Too many organic ills are, in fact, caused by years of dietary indiscretions. The modern American who has eaten improperly suddenly finds himself chronically ill—victim of one or more of the usual organic derangements: hepatitis or liver torpidity, gall or kidney stones, asthma or emphysema, coronary thrombosis or arteriosclerosis. Avoiding illness—or acquiring health—is simply a matter of hygienic everyday living.

Several Indian beliefs are relevant. The Cherokees maintained that in most cases disease results from what we eat. An ill Cherokee was instructed either to fast a few days or to abstain from salt, hot or greasy foods, and all meat. A common Choctaw belief also held that people became sick mostly from eating the wrong foods. Ethnobotanist Huron H. Smith says that while the Ojibwe "know nothing about vitamins or chemical constituents, they think that there are some salts or minerals in their native foods *that keep them well.* We know that they are correct in that. They ascribe many of their present diseases to the abandonment of their native food and the adoption of the white man's foods. They think that the early failure of their teeth is due to using too much white flour for bread."

The young people of the Hopi tend to forsake the greens and herbal foods of the old folk and turn instead to the foods of the white man: white sugar, white flour, and canned food. The Cherokees of North Carolina, too, have greatly increased the consumption of refined flour and sugar products, pastries, and other store-bought items, along with chemical drugs to palliate the ailments arising from the worsening of their health. One must realize that one does not become ill without due cause, and with very few exceptions we are all responsible for the illnesses we contract. We alone are the architects of our good health.

Herbal remedies are falling into disuse, but, while they are not intended to supplant modern medical techniques, they do offer a genuine means of maintaining health and combatting many common ailments. Especially in a time when more and more people are looking to nature and to themselves rather than to the complexities of modern technology for sources of well-being, familiarity with nature's dispensary or the "backyard drugstore" can be greatly satisfying. The study and use of our *natural* resources is, I hope, increasing. This book is but a small beginning in the renaissance of herb lore; there is a tremendous store of knowledge yet to be recovered from the past and as much to learn in the future.

I

*About
Herbal
Medicine*

1

In the Beginning

Primitive peoples, by sheer necessity, had to seek out the secrets of nature. They possessed no books, had no formal education, attended no school or college, had no other teacher or training than their direct observation of what occurred in their immediate surroundings and physical contacts. At the beginning of man's development, he was an apt student of nature, and must have noticed well the foraging of birds and animals for food-stuffs and healing remedies. These creatures instructed him which plants to select, which to avoid. And so, on an experimental basis, he might have found plants that temporarily satisfied a thirst or appetite, others that warmed his system when he felt chilled or feverish, others that rested him and, at times, made him sleepy, and some that caused not only stomach distress but, sometimes, vomiting and diarrhea. Thus, probably, did the art of healing originate.

One may reasonably assume that if our ancestors at the end of the Old Stone Age some 17,000 years ago were sufficiently cultured to create weapons and varied artifacts and tools, they also possessed the intelligence to produce the means of treating their illnesses and injuries, not only through some kind of magic or sorcery but, more important, through simple herb remedies. No doubt the ancient medicine man made sure that his incantation rituals and dances (which were actually prayers) always accompanied the administration of the therapeutic treatments, whether the drinking of herbal draughts, local applications and poultices, or steam baths; if one didn't work, the other was sure to.

As time progressed, man learned to record on stone, and afterwards on wood and papyrus, his careful observations of both wild and domestic creatures. Even today we are aware that when an animal is ill it looks for a specific medicine in nearby plants. The sick dog seeks dog-grass to effect emesis; thus the Indians would not keep an ill dog tied or shut in, so that it could find its own remedies. Grazing animals choose particular plants as healing medicine. Cats and dogs purge themselves with certain grasses, and lie in wet mud (a source of natural antibiotic) in case of snake or insect bites or other irritations. Choctaw Indians observed that the hog roots in the ground for its source of medicine.

The bear was considered to be one of the chief animals which locate sources of medicinal herbs for the healing of man. It finds plants which other animals do not notice, seeks out roots, for its claws are well adapted for digging, and is quite fond of cherries, juneberries, and acorns, all of which, together with rockberries or bearberries, have become sources of healing medicines for man as well.

Generally it has been found that those foods—grasses and roots—which animals eat are equally good for man. One of my grandfather's experiments was to watch, as did his Indian friends, the pigeons, pheasants, and partridges gather an assortment of green leaves and tender young buds of plants, and he too found these choice bits good to eat. Another experiment was undertaken several years ago by agricultural scientists to show that sheep, whose diet had been purposely deprived of calcium (lime) would go directly to the grass of a previously limed area as if led there, before visiting another plot lacking the needed mineral.

That certain plants were poisonous must have frequently

been observed by the earliest of herbalists. To this day the specifics of such observations are perpetuated in their common names. Thus an herb, because it is sometimes fatal to swine, was labeled sowbane; water hemlock is cowbane, because it is a poison to cattle. Wolf's-bane, dogbane, and henbane are other examples. Of henbane, the plant observers in the early Middle Ages noted that to eat or drink its infusion would cause madness and cause an unnatural deep sleep; thus a synonym for this herb is Insana.

Observing the reactions of wild and domestic animals to plants, the early herbalists and botanists gradually discovered the healing possibilities of local medicinal herbs. Evidently these early discoveries worked hand in hand with the practice of trial and error, and, when possible, were either tried out under the observation of trained herbalists or taken in very small doses by the laity. It is interesting that the following ancient herbal remedies offer antiseptic-healing properties for use today, either by themselves or as commercial preparations.

Centuries ago herbalists wrote about the use of the fennel plant by snakes, whose eyesight it is supposed to have restored. When about to attack a poisonous snake, a weasel was supposed to arm itself by eating a few sprigs of rue, which has long been highly valued as a remedy for the stings of all insects. The name of hawkweed is taken from falconry and was applied to the herb by the ancient Greeks, who believed that since hawks improved their sight with the plant, the herb's juice must be similarly employed in the eye complaints of humans. Pliny says that dittany's power to extract arrows was proven by the deer who, hit by such missiles, was able to loosen them by feeding on this plant. In the original seal of the Faculty of Paris, the emblem of medicine was composed of three storks with twigs of origan (wild marjoram) held in their beaks. The birds' awareness of the herb's therapeutic value was apparently widely accepted in all circles of French life.

The history and lore of herbs and herbal healing are not only the foundation of medicine; they have served as a guideline throughout history, and have outlived many cultures and civilizations. To trace the history and backgrounds of the healing arts from the early Babylonians and Egyptians through the Mosaic laws of the Hebrews and Hellenistic culture is to discover that the physicians then were true health scientists.

The Therapeutic Papyrus of Thebes, written over 3,500 years ago, maintained that the heartbeat was to be compared to the Nile's to-and-fro inundations: "There is in the heart a vessel leading to every member of the body. If the physician places his finger on the head, neck, arms, foot or body, everywhere will he find the heart, for the heart leads to every member." The Papyrus mentions approximately 700 herbal remedies, many of which still serve the medical practice, including castor and olive oils, squill, gentian, colchicum, saffron, pomegranate, hyoscyamus, coriander, and acacia.

Extensive herbal knowledge has been continually revealed throughout history. Hernando Cortes, Spanish conqueror of Mexico, discovered in the sixteenth century that the Nahuatl tribes of Mexico had for generations practiced highly scientific methods of healing and possessed a remarkable knowledge of medicinal herbs and their properties. And when they were conquered by the ruthless Spanish conquistadors, none of their European counterparts, Cortes wrote, was more skilled in remedial herbs than these Aztecs. Necessity had taught the natives of foreign lands—of South America, the East Indies, and Africa—the urgent need for a complete knowledge of herbs as well as dependency for foodstuffs and clothing material upon local flora, and so when "discovered" by whites, the natives were found to be well versed in the proper therapeutics of a surprising number of plants.

2

Superstition or Medicine?

The common, nondescript herbs or "weeds" have since time immemorial been used not only as a source of nourishment for human and beast but as remedies, dyes, and cosmetic aids. Today's discoveries of medicinal cures are the result of the observations and experiments of man throughout the ages. Each generation bequeathed its herbal findings, gained by long periods of trial and error, to the next. Discoveries were probably achieved more often by accident than by scientific experimentation, and by the slow testing and refining of folklore's original notions about herbs.

It is now becoming apparent that the use of herbs as healing remedies, long a part of the common culture throughout the world, has actually been the basis for many modern "discoveries" and "breakthroughs." Examples confirmed by laboratory tests today are the use of onions and garlic as antiseptics in diseases of the alimentary and bronchial tracts, the dandelion in liver disorders, wild sarsaparilla as a detoxifier of the bloodstream, lovage and masterwort as cleaners of the alimentary and intestinal canals, and the stems of cinquefoil and gold thread as an application to torn skin wounds and ulcers. The unsaturated oil of safflower is today employed in medicine for jaundice and malfunctions of the gallbladder, although such use originated in folklore which read the "signature" for this very application in the orange-red flowers and the yellow coloring matter of the herb.

Are herbal remedies superstition or medicine? Beneath every so-called superstition there may be an as yet undisclosed truth. I think of herbal remedies in the dictionary sense of "folklore," as "the traditional beliefs, legends, and customs of a (or of the common) people," noting that "lore" is defined as "a body of knowledge, especially of a traditional, anecdotal, or popular nature, on a particular subject." Our parents and grandparents, often without formal schooling, were knowledgeable and competent people. They relied upon the store of information handed down through the ages for a variety of needs, including simple remedies, and seemed to do quite well without the advice of experts for every sneeze and twinge.

Each people, each country has its favorite herbal remedy. The Chinese have used huge quantities of ginseng root to restore vitality. Chamomile is the favored treatment in Germany and Scandinavian countries for colds and stomach ailments. The forest yielded the West Indians a time-tested remedy, mauby bark, against anemia, and ginger root against colds. Americans in the Southern states are especially fond of a blood-purifying beverage made from sassafras bark. There are myriad Hungarian gypsy herbal treatments: the leaves of the sweet chestnut for asthmatic complaints, cleavers or parsley piert for bladder trouble, stinging nettle for blood pressure and for softening hardened arteries, rosemary for stimulating the hair follicles and scalp, cranesbill root for diarrhea, milkweed for pleurisy.

Several years ago, a London news report headlined "Witches' Potions Superior to Many Modern Medicines Says British Physician" stated: "It is revealed that more and more doctors are recommending herbal treatment for their patients. Recent scientific investigation has shown that herbal prescriptions, once regarded as 'old wives' tales,' are actually beneficial. . . . 'Old wives' tales' which have proved their merit include [the following]. Sphagnum moss has been used for centuries by Irish peasants. During the World War it was discovered to be preferable to lint for dressing. . . . For inflamed eyes, the best remedy is a leek pounded to pulp and applied to the eyes between muslin pads. . . . A potion of boiled laurels and ivy leaves is invaluable for burns and scalds. . . . The juice of the celandine shrivels warts. . . . The Irish cure their colds in a few hours by eating a jelly made by boiling a species of seaweed with a field flower."

I myself was initiated at a very early age into the drinking of healthful herb teas. I still recall my grandfather holding a cup of recently brewed herb tea and his command, "Drink!" I drank a cupful upon rising and another before bedtime. And this bitter brew has sweetened the writer's health for over sixty years. Each fall and winter called for such cold-preventers, or "fever chasers," as Grandfather called them, as catnip, mint, boneset, yarrow, and purple verbena; the "spring (blood-cleanser) tonic" consisted principally of burdock, dandelion, sassafras, and sarsaparilla. Today, in turn, I am known for my herb teas in my own family.

It is from the healing lore of all peoples, of almost every part of the world, that much of our medical treatments and materia medica are derived. Physical therapy has long been known to and practised by the lay healers of Japan, China, and India: moxa was employed by the Japanese and, with acupuncture, by the Chinese (the latter also wore spectacles in the fifteenth century) ; inoculation was a common practice of the Hindus, Persians, and Chinese as was hypnotism by the Hindus. The North American Indians had a worthy substitute for the Turkish or Swedish bath, their vapor baths, in their local hot springs or geysers and in the sweat-oven. Usually the strange "herb-women" of foreign lands turned out to be the wise women of unblemished repute who practiced specialties of herb therapy and midwifery, a well-known combination in common practice until the twenties of this century.

As for herbal therapeutics, a glance at the healing methods

of old rural England shows that the remedies of the past are
still very much in use today: dandelion, chamomile, and mint
for stomach disorders, wormwood and gentian as systemic ton-
ers and stimulants, colchicum (meadow saffron) for gout, hoarhound and marsh mallow for coughs and colds, male fern for
worms, and fennel and eyebright for impaired eyesight. Modern medicine has derived from the aborigines' fatal arrow poisons such life-saving drugs a ouabin, curare, and veratrin. Our
Indian medicine men regarded the following as examples of
their vast treasure of healing herbs: sassafras and sarsaparilla
for purifying the bloodstream, lobelia for asthmatic coughs,
wild cherry and sumac for relief of sore throat and colds, and
willow for rheumatic pains. Only with the help of the Quebec
Iroquois could Jacques Cartier, the French navigator, in the
years 1535 and 1536, treat the ravages of scurvy in his crew so
very successfully with fresh infusions of the leaves and bark of
the hemlock spruce. The cinchona of the Peruvian Indians became the physician's specific against malarial fever, which for
centuries had baffled the most learned of the medical profession.
Digitalis, the English herb-woman's famous remedy, was eventually administered by Dr. William Withering to his dropsy or
cardiac patients. Rauwolfia is now prescribed for high blood
pressure, and sarsaparilla for blood disorders. Folklore was
also instrumental in developing a "new" concept in preventative
medicine: that a simple, basic diet of native uncooked vegetables and fruits and daily drinks of herb teas prevented not only
scurvy but a host of ailments.

Even medical doctors, when disillusioned with chemical
drugs, have tested herb remedies and found them as effective as
standard prescription drugs. (In fact, I found during my more
than thirty years as a druggist that many newly-arrived foreign
physicians would frequently recommend prescriptions composed
only of herbal ingredients and as often would prefer my own
preparations to factory-made patent remedies.) Ambroise Paré,
the French surgeon of the sixteenth century, for instance, is re-

ported to have carried on such herbal experiments. At one time, when pressed for a fast-acting remedy for fresh, severe burns, he adopted a friend's treatment, raw slices of onion. To the one burned cheek of the patient he applied the onion, to the other the standard lotion of the day, and found the onion remedy far more efficacious. Present-day physicians often suggest a soothing cream for skin irritations that is prepared from castor oil, zinc oxide, and corn starch. Watermelon has been medically prescribed for a number of kidney disorders, with satisfying results.

Mold poultices represent a well-known folk remedy. In Mexico the Indian women and the other economically deprived people have combatted an external infection simply by applying a "penicillin" mold which had formed on a tortilla to the affected area. My grandfather used bread mold and his Indian cohorts various leaf molds. In China it was believed that eating bits of "dragon bones" would drive away the evil spirits that caused fits in babies. These bones were actually the bones of dinosaurs found buried in the Gobi desert, and were quickly utilized as a food and as a source of the easily absorbed mineral calcium, which is so often prescribed by today's doctors for nervous and muscular (convulsive) disorders of babies. In the early 1800s, the ashes of burnt sponges were recommended by herbalists for neck swellings. Half a century later the dried sea animal became officially accepted by the medical profession as *Spongeia usta* and prescribed for goiter (or swelling of the neck) because of its high content of iodine and other minerals.

Let us determine how new "discoveries" are come by in the medical or drug manufacturer's laboratory. If research may be defined as the systematic investigation of a given subject so that facts or principles may be discovered, then the modern researcher's own findings and analyses are but the tip of the iceberg. Today's medical researchers must industriously study the folk remedies of various lands for clues which may lead to "new" drug products. In 1970 a project for this very purpose was jointly undertaken by members of the American Society of Pharmacognosy and members of American Doctors. These men volunteered for assignments in city and backwoods hospitals and clinics in Central and South America, the Far East, Southeast Asia, and Africa to observe and evaluate folkloric remedies.

Since 1943 investigators have found that many familiar herbs and table foods, various plant parts and their extracts have decidedly therapeutic virtues which very often contain pronounced antibiotic agents. Among them are the lotus, olive, laurel, myrtle, and garlic, used as remedies by the Assyrians; dates, figs, crocus, opium, onion, and lettuce, used by the Egyptians; the extracts and juices of celery, asparagus, cabbage, pepper, and parsley, favored by the Greeks and Romans; manna, pepper, clove, camphor, croton oil, nux vomica, rhubarb, and nutmeg, recommended by the Arabian physicians. From such plants and others to which earlier literature had attributed remarkable cures, researchers at various universities, private institutes, and state agricultural experiment stations have isolated a long list of "new" and newly-named substances which have proven to be strongly antiseptic or possessing actively antibiotic or antifungal activity.

Thus have herbal medicines run the gamut from the early seemingly "magic" potions to the druggist's pills. From the herbs of the fields and marshes, from our fruits and vegetables (which up to two centuries ago were known as herbs), from molds and fungi and lichens, from trees and cultivated garden flowers and ornamentals, indeed, from all vegetation of sea and land have come modern medical "discoveries."

3

The American Indians

The remarkable contribution which the American Indian has made to American culture, including its healing practices, need not be relegated to the forgotten past. His keen insight regarding the selective uses of native plants produced nutritious food, beverages, and effective healing agents, as well as an assortment of dyes, mats and baskets, cords and string of various thicknesses, canoes, and many household artifacts.

Our early American history books were full of grossly mistaken though widely held images of the Indian. That very name often conjured up to youthful readers a mighty warrior, terrible tales of raids, scalping parties, and assorted bloody acts. But his peaceful side was ill reported. In truth, we owe much to the Indians. The first Thanksgiving proclamation given out by Massachusetts Governor Bradford in 1621 really should be dedicated to the original natives who taught the newly arrived Europeans how to stave off hunger not only with weedlike edibles and easily trapped wild life, but with vegetable foodstuffs cultivated in their gardens. The settlers on the James River in Virginia were long hungry in the midst of plenty until their dark-skinned teachers taught them that the "hard shells"— oysters—were a source of nourishment.

The white colonists obtained much valuable knowledge from their red friends and soon acquired the Indian arts of canoeing, tobogganing, and snowshoeing, as well as techniques of snaring birds and animals and obtaining a large supply of fish without the customary hook and pole, all of which foods were herb-seasoned with aromatics at hand's reach and found pleasant to the taste and digestion. And, furthermore, the white men learned from their Indian instructors certain methods of agriculture—of hoeing and planting of seeds in hills, of fertilizing the vegetable patches, of weeding out plants but later employing them in many useful ways, of interplanting corn with beans or squash, of protecting the corn-field with a scarecrow and preserving the unshelled food in a corn-crib.

After their first contact with the Indians, the white men discovered Indian agriculture, which, despite the lack of familiar Old World plants, was quite sophisticated. The experience of these knowledgeable natives—and their generosity—prevented a frightful food shortage for the white pioneers. We can thank these Amerind gardeners for pone, hominy, succotash, and of course maple syrup and breads made from the cambium layers of that tree. Today, people still think of agriculture in connection with so-called "civilized" culture and of Indians as eating only wild foods. But they, as well as the aborigines of South America, had developed cultivation of food plants to a much higher degree than had the newly arrived whites. The Aztecs, Incas, and Mayas established their society on corn, of which plentiful harvests provided them with profit and leisure to create remarkable cultures. Indians of both Americas grew this great botanical mystery, which cannot reproduce itself in the wild state, but is a most nutritious member of the grass family. The Wisconsin Potawatomi and the Pueblo Indians of the Southwest were noted for their agriculture, and the Choctaws have well earned their title, "a nation of farmers." Not only did they excel all North American Indians in this area, they subsisted largely on the products of their cultivated fields.

Many of the Indians' crops are quite familiar. Maize and panic species were powdered and made into bread, which also contained powdered sunflower seeds. Their vegetables included leeks, garlic, and cabbage, and they harvested huge amounts of beans (*Phaseolus*), hyacinth beans (*Dolichos*), and sweet potatoes. Squash grew in abundance as did the Indians' Jerusalem artichokes and assorted melons. Not only did the varieties of gourds serve as foodstuff; they provided serviceable household wares like cups, dippers, and other vessels. Other cultivated plants of the New World residents included the white potato, strawberry, tomato, lima beans, peanut, cacao, chili pepper, manioc (tapioca), and avocado (the latter in warmer climates).

To augment his vegetable produce, the Indian took advantage of fresh and salt water fish, which served a twofold purpose as food and fertilizer. For the latter purpose, the coastal Indians tucked one of the easily snared alewives into each hill of corn as it was planted. The abundant wild turkey, deer, bear, and other familiar animals; the nuts, obviously a foodstuff saved for winter use—hickory, acorn, hazelnut, black walnut and the now extinct chestnut—and the dozens of fruits which were eaten fresh or dried for times of food scarcity—blackberries, blueberries, chokeberries, grapes, plums, and especially cranberries—all of these claimed their niche in the natives' larder. Of the wild-growing, weedy food plants, there were fresh vegetable greens, which were also included in soups or stews, or combined with other cooked vegetables, or dried and preserved for the winter months.

Many of the edible native plants discovered by the American Indian yielded gradual alterative, non-visible efforts; others provided more obvious therapeutic results: they either acted upon the kidneys or intestines or helped to heal some organic ailment. Thus from early childhood he was intimate with scores of remedial herbs and each of these he would accurately identify with a given disease.

First hand information regarding Indian healing pursuits and everyday life is difficult to obtain, as I discovered when in

1955 I visited a Seminole group in Florida. What little was disclosed to me was known generally and offered nothing new. The Indians are justifiably reluctant to discuss or part with their hard-earned, cherished knowledge. Having divulged it long ago to the thankless white newcomers, they were soon to be cut off from their food supply and forced to live in barren concentration camps—the reservations—amidst humiliating poverty and squalor. One can hardly blame the Indian for wishing he had not been so friendly.

Perhaps the most striking legacy of the Indian is his vast knowledge of medicinal plants and their therapeutic properties. His excellent knowledge of hundreds of plants was obtained, not from college professors, but from first hand, practical experience. Scores of plant derivatives identified by the Indian were later to be included in such official compendia as the *United States Pharmacopoeia* and the *National Formulary* and employed by modern medical practitioners. The Indians were never at a loss to recognize the herb indicated to heal a particular ailment, and the time of year it was to be collected. And not only was their knowledge of medicinal plants considerable, but equally outstanding was their comprehensive practice of various healing treatments, of surgery and mid-wifery. They operated "with a skill," according to O. Phelps Brown, an American herbal physician of over a century ago, "that far surpasses many a learned doctor of the big medical schools, with all their science, and the medical teachings of physicians for upwards of four thousand years."

"The earth is our mother" was a favorite saying of the herb-minded North American Indian. An exceptionally observant student of nature, he memorized the many details pertaining to plants eaten by the animals; what nourished and healed the wildlife of field and forest was found to be quite safe and beneficial in most instances for him as well. He noted the rudimentary healing practices engaged in by animals, which when suffering from wounds, internal disturbances, and fever, would gather their own proper medicines. A wild turkey, for instance, during the rainy season force-feeds her little ones with the leaves of spicebush; a dog with a digestive problem chews upon the witch grass to provoke vomiting; the bear feeds upon the fruit of the rockberry with relish while fern roots become his healing agent; the wolf, bitten by a venomous snake, seeks out and chews snakeroot.

Plants, shrubs, and trees were sacred to the Ojibwe and could be gathered only with an accompanying prayer and the observance of a proper ancient ceremony. This consisted of special explanatory songs and an offering of tobacco to Grandmother Earth, to Winabojo, their cultural hero, and to the ruler of the universe. The herb-gatherers addressed their prayers to the Apportioner, the chief deity, and asked humbly for permission to come and obtain the medicine. The Indian did not ruthlessly tear up plant life. He paid, Alice Lounsberry said, "the tribute of a man's understanding to these mute inhabitants of the forests." A short prayer chant of New England Algonquians began, "Nikomo (Mother Earth), I am putting my hand into thy side to get this herb." The herb was then named three times followed by a thrice recited uttering of the plant's intended use.

The legacy of remedial herbs bequeathed to us by the Indian has served well in recent and present-day medicine. Many of the effective vegetable drugs which have been employed by the American medical practitioner for over two hundred years originated in primitive and folk medicine. A few examples will suffice:

LOBELIA	Expectorant in asthma and bronchitis
CASCARA SAGRADA	Tonic laxative
CINCHONA	Source of quinine; a bitter tonic, antimalarial
EPHEDRA	Source of ephedrine employed in bronchial asthma, hay fever, and circulatory collapse
SARSAPARILLA	Alterative in rheumatic and blood disorders

BURDOCK   Diaphoretic, diuretic, and alterative
DANDELION   Bitter and mild laxative in jaundice and
                   liver disorders
MANDRAKE   A cholagogue cathartic in liver and gall-
                   bladder disorders
JUNIPER   Stimulant, aromatic, and diuretic
GOLDENSEAL   A strong alterative for gastro-intestinal
                   and nasal catarrh
GENTIAN   Bitter tonic in digestive disturbances and
                   dyspepsia
DIGITALIS   Diuretic and cardiac stimulant
PYRETHRUM   Insecticide and parasiticide
SQUILL   Expectorant, diuretic, cardiac stimulant
OPIUM   Source of morphine, codeine; somnifa-
                   cient, calmative, and analgesic
LICORICE   Demulcent and expectorant
ELM   Demulcent and emollient

Further contributions to American medicine are the Aztecs'
age-old employment of such well-known plants as cochineal,
stramonium, passion flower, cotton, liquidambar, and the con-
troversial tobacco; the Mayas' capsicum (red pepper), guaiac,
vanilla, and chenopodium; and the coca, ipecac, and curare of
the South American Indians.

Often, however, Indian medicine has been ignored or re-
jected as worthless until its later "discovery" in the laboratory.
A case in point is the Amerind's use of oral contraceptives.
In the beginning, the medicine man recommended gromwell
as a diuretic to enhance the removal of stone formations from
the kidneys, and based his judgement on the plant's appearance
—the stony-hard, egg-shaped seeds (thus the generic name,
Lithospermum)—and its habitat of dry, gravelly soil. Eventually, the Indian women of the Northwestern states who had
been drinking the herb brew for several weeks, and up to six
months, may have reported their failure to conceive. Eventually

this long-concealed discovery was laboratory-tested for contraceptive possibilities. The researchers found that an extract of the plant completely nullified the normally recurring physiological changes of the female sexual organ. Another extract tested upon laboratory animals produced a marked decrease in the number of estrous smears, and, on rats, reduced ovarian gonadotropism.

After generations of almost continual food scarcity, resulting principally from the greed of the white wasters of game and cultivatable lands, and destroyers of field and forest, the Indians resorted to the practice of birth control as the only means of reducing overpopulation and food consumption, a concept which has been widely advocated in our time. Thus strong infusions of gromwell by the Shoshone women were used as a trustworthy contraceptive, and of wild geranium by the Nevadan mother of a month-old infant to provide her with an approaching pregnancy-safe year. To provide temporary sterility, concentrated infusions of the following plants were taken: dogbane (*Apocynum androsaemifolium*), milkweed (*Asclepias syrica* and species), antelope sage (*Eriogonum jamesii*) and deer's tongue (*Frasera speciosa*). To a limited degree, the combined boiled leaves of Solomon's seal and juniper berries, the boiled roots of mountain hollyhock and the infused freshly collected root of false hellebore (*Adonis* species) were also used.

The relationship that existed between the tribal healers and their patients was an enviable one, especially according to today's standards. This feature is clearly emphasized by the cooperative healing practices of two distinct groups: the medicine man and woman, i.e. the "physicians," and the local shaman.

The shaman was called the "mystery man (or woman)," the "singer," or "chanter" and was generally credited with working wonders through interpretations of dreams and the recognition and removal of the more mysterious (perhaps psychosomatic) causes of illnesses. While the prayer-songs were recited in the presence of the ailing one to help drive away or frighten the evil spirits which were supposedly tormenting him (this was "white magic," as opposed to "black magic" which brought disease and misfortune upon a tribe's enemies), the shaman's therapy often became most effective through the power of suggestion.

Such therapy was conducted in close cooperation with the Indian "physician," who was a most competent botanist, herbalist, and naturalist. His education, in some ways, was more rigorous than our modern medical school. He was required to "pass" a fully detailed, years-long course composed of all aspects of the healing procedures as taught by a skilled teacher-doctor. His character had to be impeccable: if he was known to be lazy, careless, quarrelsome, or jealous, he would not be favorably received. Along with learning to accurately diagnose and treat a given variety of illnesses with several given compound preparations, he was also required to master the complete lore of sacred incantations, love conjuring, hunting and fishing formulas, ritual bathing practices, and so on. For four to seven successive days he drank a decoction of herbs—pitcher plant, burdock, black birch, golden alexander and others—to help him remember his newly acquired knowledge. He was taught that every tree, herb, and bush offered some good, purposeful use, and in time, he, too, became a repository of herbal knowledge. But he considered his plant remedies as unique, so that when questioned about them, he invariably repeated the often-heard words of his tutor: "I can tell you about my own medicines. I do not know about other peoples' medicines nor their uses of the same plants." (Quite often other tribes had different names and medicinal uses for the same herb.) And in manner similar to our physician's need to properly identify the various symptoms and arrive at a correct diagnosis of the patient's illness, so, too, was the Indian doctor ably qualified to analyze the symptoms and the causes of the disorder. However, it should be noted that the medicine man, upon healing the sick, by whatever measures, took no credit for such accomplishments

but reminded his patients that all knowledge and power of healing came from spirits; the origin of such restoration to health
was readily accepted as supernatural.

Like the Israelites and Egyptians and their neighbors who
burned incense and aromatic oils in their temples, the Indians
engaged in crude fumigations whose vapors would drive away
the sickness-causing evil spirits. Rising heavenward, the acrid
smoke of evergreens—cypress, for example—and strongly
scented plants was intended to dispel malicious influences upon
health.

To the Indians this singular feature of healing, the sweat
bath, served not only as a sanitary expedient, it became a remedy
for nearly all disorders, whatever their seriousness, for children
with chicken pox and for the elders with rheumatism. The
favorite remedy of the Aztecs for nearly all their ills was their
vapor-bath or *temazcalli*. The Indians of eastern Pennsylvania,
South and North Carolina, and especially New Mexico, held
the therapeutic values of warm mineral springs in high esteem.
The waters were used as an internal cleanser, a treatment for
rheumatic disorders and other chronic maladies, and externally
for ulcers, tetters, itch, and other skin problems. Among the
countless reports by settlers which noted the plant lore of the
early Amerinds, one related the healing of William Bratton,
a member of the Lewis-Clark Northwest expedition, through a
sweat bath treatment. He had suffered for months almost un-
bearable back pains and rheumatic stiffness which prevented him
from riding or walking. All the customary medicines prescribed
by his white colleagues having failed, a kind of Indian steam
bath was prepared by pouring water over hot stones in Indian
style. Bratton also drank the required strong hot infusion of
horsemint, and after a few treatments of this combination, the
explorer is reported to have recovered so completely that he
was able to resume active duties.

A religious rite was engaged in prior to a Cherokee patient's
entrance to the sweat-lodge. He sipped a sudorific (sweat-

causing) herb potion or chewed an aromatic root while the
medicine man gently rubbed his forehead and sang a prayer-
song of healing, an incantation of holy words believed to give
the entire herbal treatment greater efficacy. And just as today's
clergymen, psychiatrists, and psychologists can influence the
patient's mental attitude, the medicine man caused his patient
to believe he was getting well.

The Indians claim that many of the medicinal plants which
they employ for healing purposes are received in dreams. It is
quite likely that the "dream" may have occurred to the medicine
man during a lengthy meditation following a customary fast of
a few days or while in a secluded "retreat" in the religious or
spiritual sense.

On his first visit to the patient, the medicine man evaluated
all the possible clues and symptoms, asked many questions. He
then retired to his "office" where he meditated in a restful position, the better to complete the "dream" in which the diagnosis
and remedy for the ailment are sought.

The medicine man was careful to treat the whole person, not
just a particular organ or one part of the body, for the whole
body was affected, dysfunctioning, when one was troubled with
a feverish cold or deep bronchial cough, or with rheumatic aches
or painful stone formations.

One approach to temporary ailment was to rub the patient's
abdomen four times and make him drink a strong herb decoction
to cause quick vomiting. If the ailment was of a more severe
and lasting nature, the patient underwent the sweat-bath treatment. And if the condition still continued, the patient was isolated ("hospitalized") and underwent a few days of fasting.
The medicine man imposed a fast upon himself as well for the
first complete day while treating the patient.

At no time was the Cherokee patient allowed any salt or
salted foods, fatty meats, peppers and other spicy articles, or
cooked foods. In diarrhea cases, chicken and fish were forbidden, as was milk in urinary conditions; and in rheumatism, the

patient was forbidden to eat buffalo fish, sun perch, squirrel and buffalo. (Today flesh foods are forbidden to arthritics because of their uric acid content.)

The medicine man, having decided upon the nature of the illness, now proceeded to prescribe a specific remedy. Of the many items constituting American Indian materia medica, the greater number were unquestionably derived from the plant kingdom, of which the majority were fresh or dried roots and entire plants, although barks, stems, flowers, leaves, fruits, and seeds were also employed. To a much lesser degree, a few animal and mineral drugs were used. The Indians' preparations included infusions (teas), liniments, plasters, ointments, lotions, and especially decoctions.

Long before the arrival of the early colonists, the medicine men had already been prescribing a wide variety of preparations: cathartics and diuretics, alteratives, emetics, cough and cold remedies, astringents, vermifuges, antiseptics, and narcotics. And while admittedly they did not know the full pharmacological nature of their medications, they were satisfied with the effects which resulted from the prescribed medicine. Years of attentive observation and a well experienced, trial-and-error practice made results predictable and side-effects unlikely. (The modern physician is well aware of the many "side effects, contraindications, adverse reactions, warnings and precautions" which accompany prescribed drugs.) Too often, however, the cures of the Indian practitioner were discredited by the whites simply because his methods and treatment routine included the ceremonial chanting and dance. Dr. Benjamin Rush, the eminent Revolutionary physician of Philadelphia, on his first acquaintance with Indian medicine said, "We have no discoveries in the materia medica to hope for from the Indians of North America." But only a few years later, upon hearing the reports of his colleagues, he admitted to a high regard for indigenous medicines. Not only did the Indian teach the pioneering white men much about their newly adopted surroundings and various means of overcoming the hardships of a new, strange country, he often prevented an early demise of many of their sick by treating them with nearby herbs as well as indicating to the healed which plants to use as preventative medicine.

Because there was no single vocabulary for the commonly used herbs, since the names varied from one tribe to another, the Indian herbalist offered original designations of known plants and trees. At times the same name was given to several plants and often one plant would have several names, as here noted. Even an individual other than an herbalist, herb-collector, or medicine-man could have a pet name for a remedial herb. Thus, the Chippewa, for instance, designated names of plants which usually were compound nouns; and these nouns, in turn, indicated the place where it grew, the appearance of the plant, its principal use or characteristic property. In addition, a suffix indicated which part of the plant was employed, such as the leaf, the root, or the flower. (And indeed that was how the candidate for the office of medicine man studied herb-lore.)

To the self-taught students of nature, the herbalists and healers of the American Indians, symbolism and sympathetic principles were inseparable from their diagnoses and remedies. Here are a few examples of plants and their "signatures" which led to their designation for specific uses, as indicated by the medicine men of different tribes:

PIÑON, *Pinus edulis,* "gum branch." The synonym indicates the tree's high yield of a gummy exudation. This substance was much employed in infrequent micturation, kidney disorders, and syphilis. An open skin infection or ulcer was covered with piñon gum to effect quicker healing.

GOLDENROD, *Solidago canadensis,* "inside flower seeds." The name is an allusion to the seeds in the blossom. An infusion of the blossoms was taken several times a day to relieve "inside" pains of the body.

SARSAPARILLA, *Aralia racemosa* and *A. nudicalis,* "legs."

These valued roots were employed as alteratives in blood poisoning and as a poultice to reduce inflammatory swellings and infections on legs and arms.

MILKWEED, *Asclepias syriaca,* "milk." This plant exemplifies an associated or symbolic therapy. The milk of this plant resembled mother's milk and therefore was served to treat or prevent faulty lactation, a practice still engaged in by Indian women, especially the Tewas of the New Mexico Pueblos. Although the plant served at first as a "female remedy," the Ojibwe also ate the fresh flowers and tips in soups or cooked them with meats, those herbal parts then becoming of a mucilaginous consistency, which led to their employment as a diaphoretic-expectorant in pleurisy, asthma, and other catarrhal disorders of the bronchia.

WILD GINGER, *Asarum canadense,* "sturgeon potato" or "ginger." This "hot" potato became a favorite remedy in acute febrile infections and a much-used diaphoretic and carminative for colds and stomach colic.

Ferns served a double purpose. The Cherokee medicine man placed great remedial value in several species of ferns as antirheumatics because the unrolling of the fronds suggests the straightening out of contracted muscles and limbs. Rheumatism, it was said, was caused by the measure worm, the cramped movements of the patient resembling those of the worm. (This is the theory behind the use of other ferns as worm expellants.) Early European herbalists, as well, employed a decoction of the fresh root of the common oak fern or dried powders of it for rheumatic swellings of the joints. John Gerard, the sixteenth-century English herbalist, states that in previous centuries, especially amongst Arabian physicians of the period 900–1100 A.D., these ferns were often credited as a specific remedy in arthritis and in aches of the joints. He further states that "Dioscorides saith that the root of Polypodie [fern] is very good for members out of joint." However, the young, uncurled fronds of several ferns, especially the male fern, *Dryopteris filix-mas,* and the lady fern, *Asplenium filix-femina,* resembled curled-up snakes and thus led the ancients and Indian doctors to use these plants as worm expellants.

The red color of herbs indicated their power of healing the blood, internally and externally. Of the red dock and related species, a poultice of the leaves was applied to scorbutic areas, ulcers, and especially to fresh wounds. (The sixteenth-century English *Ascham's Herbal* informs us that the ashes of these burnt leaves "fretteth away dead flesh of a wound.") An infusion of the leaves and roots, taken several times a day, yielded its deobstruent, blood-cleansing, and detergent properties.

If roses were red, then to the Chippewa medicine man red signified the bloodstream; the reddish flowers and fruits (hips) of the herb were to be consumed as a foodstuff and as a tea. A weak infusion of the flowers helped greatly to soothe irritated or bloodshot eyes. Other eclectic practitioners placed thin scrapings or a powder of the stem within the wound and bandaged it, with the amazing result that there seldom remained even the least trace of a scar. Various species of rose possess decided antibiotic as well as astringent properties.

The Indian herb gatherer recognized the roughly spotted and lenticelled barks of elder and sumac as healing agents with which he prepared decoctions and ointments to apply to all affections of the skin, which is the "bark" or outer covering of the body.

All shrubs and trees which yielded gums, balsams, or resins were indicated as healing agents for open and infected sores, wounds, and ulcers.

Burdock and pitcher plant were especially valued for their power to enable the candidate medicine man not only to acquire knowledge but to remember all he had learned. To keep the acquired knowledge "sticking in the mind" while he fasted for four to seven days, he must drink a brew of burdock (or varieties of bur plants) since burs themselves stick and cling to whatever comes in contact with them. Also esteemed as a memoryretaining herb, the leaves of the pitcher plant offered a ready-made liquid which was consumed by the applicant. The theory was that since the leaves kept entrapped all insects and other things that had fallen into them, this plant served also to keep in the mind the knowledge acquired.

Slippery elm's bark was employed when something was to be ejected from the body, either from the bronchia or in childbirth. The idea was to make the inside slippery by using the sap and juice (or a decoction) of the tree's bark, which are of a mucilaginous character.

Sourwood, *Oxydendrum arboreum,* has been employed even recently by physicians as a powerful diuretic, especially in dropsy and in feverish conditions, and by Indian doctors in a prescription against the suppression of the urine. To bring quick relief, he chose this herb, with its smooth, even twigs, to restore the urinary passages, thought to be twisted, coiled, and obstructed by disease, to their original straight, smooth condition.

Shrubs which have their roots in water—hydrangea, sycamore, and alder—were to be employed in urinary disorders and related ailments. The medicine men advanced the explanation that the unobstructed contact of these roots with water rendered a greater effectiveness in the treatment of organs whose liquid (such as urine or blood) was afflicted with disorder.

There are other interesting Indian remedies. The female members of the Andean tribes partook of dried eggs of salt water fish to increase and insure their fertility. But every tribal member as well ate this food for a different purpose, as a source of iodine. From their years of experience came this accurate and sensible explanation for eating the fish eggs—so that they would not be afflicted with the "big necks [goiter] of the whites." Now modern physicians prescribe oral solutions of iodine for goiter and lay folk take tablets of sea-weed or kelp, which, unlike the prescription liquid iodine, contain *all* of the ocean's major and trace minerals.

To prevent "souring of the stomach," the Quechuas, who were related to the Incas, immersed potatoes in a water suspension of a white clay, which may have appeared utterly outlandish to the visiting investigator. Again there was a rational explanation. The clay, containing traces of an aromatic, vanilla-like substance, coumarin, consisted principally of a mineral called kaolin (aluminum silicate), which has only recently been introduced into several drugstore remedies. The therapeutic properties of this material depend upon its ability to protect the mucosa of the stomach and intestines from poisonous substances and from bacterial toxins, thus its frequent internal use in the treatment of gastro-enteritis and infectious dysentery. (A similar folk practice of "earth eating" [geophagy] was common among the poor of Louisiana, Mississippi, and other southern states. They occasionally ate pieces of washed clay which they said acted as a "general regulator," made them feel good, and "purified the blood.")

From the American Indian, the whites learned that the oft-cited ounce of prevention should be heeded at each meal, by consuming fresh fruits, vegetables (some cooked), whole grain cereals and grains, and a minimum of overcooked meats or fish.

When Dr. Weston Price visited the Indians of the Yukon Territory in 1933, he was told that scurvy was a "white man's disease." His Indian informant admitted that some of his people could succumb to scurvy but at least they knew how to prevent that condition while the whites did not. (Of course, once faced with starvation, reservation Indians were forced to eat the manufactured, nutritionless, health-wasting foods of modern man. The Indians therefore must suffer the ravages of many organic disorders along with scurvy, resulting from a diet of worthless, high-caloried "empty foods.") Dr. Price discovered that one of the scurvy-preventing secrets of the

Yukon Indians was in their selection of a meat-food, as in the case of a recently killed moose. Once opened up, the two balls located in the fat of the back part were scooped out and divided evenly among the participants. By eating not only this portion but the walls of the second stomach, the Indians obtained a sufficient quantity of vitamin C from the adrenal glands and organs, considered by modern science as the most valuable source of vitamin C found in animal tissue.

From a consideration of the dietary habits of the early Canadian Indians, one discovers that they eschewed the use of salt, the white commercial kind, and harsh spices such as pepper and mustard. The "salt" with which they seasoned their bread and soups was usually the alkaline ashes of plants, natural salt licks, or the calcined bones of animals. Their seasoning herbs included various mints, wild ginger, corn silk, several species of berries, wild rice, woodbine, and the blossoms of local foods. With the coming of the profit-hungry white traders and their political allies-in-crime, the use of salt among the Chippewa became a matter of law. There was a stipulation in the infamous "Salt Treaty" of 1847 that the Indians "should receive 5 barrels of salt annually for five years." But the enterprising Amerinds had their own sources of natural salt licks, where they say "salt comes up from the ground," having been deposited on the surface by almost continual evaporation of the soil water. They had learned to live well without the addition of the synthetic, health-destroying chemical, as had the Eskimos, long after the advent of the white man. Could the taboo have resulted because salt makes meat swell, and therefore could also do the same to flesh? Or perhaps the dietary restriction arose from a different direction. James Mooney observed that "the smarting of salt in open wounds and the scalding effect of hot food have probably given the people the notion that these two articles of diet are of a pain-aggravating nature."

Among the matters of particular health importance, one takes especial note of the Indians' segregating or quarantining themselves when severely ill in a "hospital," be it hut or wigwam, for a period of four to seven days; if ailing mildly or temporarily out of sorts, the patients ate rather sparingly or restricted their food intake to water or herb tea. Further regard is taken of the Arikaras, the "corn-eaters" of the upper Missouri River, whose expectant mothers and recently delivered women adhered to prescribed diets, eating simple, wholesome foods but much less before and after the time of delivery. The pregnant woman was cautioned that excessive eating will produce a fat and over-sized baby which will needlessly increase the severity of the labor pains. After delivery, the convalescent was allowed a light broth made of vegetables or of corn, which, being easy to digest, increased the flow of milk for the infant.

There are many other examples of Indian herbal aids to health and remedies for ailments. This discussion should suffice, however, to show how varied and extensive their medicinal resources have been, and how great a contribution they have made to our culture.

4

The Doctrine of Signatures

There are several ways of learning the values of edible and medicinal plants. You can peruse botanical and anthropological tomes, or you can enroll in a class of applied botany offered by a university or an adult evening course, or you may ask interminable questions of a practicing herbalist. Or you may enter a rewarding acquaintanceship with dozens of nondescript "weeds" by learning in the field the various characteristics and peculiarities of these plants, their mode of growth, the assorted designs of their leaves, stems, or roots, colors of the flowers, and their habitat.

I use the approach described in this chapter, derived directly from the ancient doctrine of signatures, and have found it an effective teaching device. Unlike the Chippewa instruction in medicine, in which the name of the medicinal herb was secretly handed down from the Indian teacher to the pupil from generation to generation, the Western method relies on identification by name—the colloquial or common name, and the scientific Latin designation. The quickest and most effective teaching tool is the field trip. There the student can see and touch individual specimens, and closely observe the plant's habitat. Instead of tedious memorization of the various uses of a plant, the doctrine of signatures offers in many (though not all) cases a reliable system of connecting the herb with its remedial use through symbolic association.

Does the plant grow in swampy or muck soil? Then that plant might help remove hardened mucus from the ailing body. The color of this plant's flower is yellow? Then, generally, its therapeutic properties are directed toward the liver and gall-bladder. Herbs with hollow stems are indicated as cleansers of the human hollow tubes, alimentary and bronchial; others that display sharp thorns or spines are indicated as relief for sharp pains. Those that are intensely bitter to the taste should remind one of the following rule: bitter to the taste is sweet to the stomach, sweet to the taste is bitter to the stomach.

The doctrine of signatures is probably the earliest system of applied therapeutics in the history of medicine. When the earliest of herbalists associated a characteristic of plants with some part of the human anatomy, a system of herbal remedies had begun. Paracelsus based his "signatures" not only on the shapes and colors of medicine-yielding plants but upon the popular astrological notion that each signature depended upon the position of the stars. This concept was held by the sixteenth and seventeenth century herbalists Gerard and Culpepper and persists even today among some astrologers, who borrow from those herbalists their page-filling material.

However, again and again we do find countless examples of medicinal herbs on which are "stamped" an indication of their healing properties. The inquisitive novice herbalist need only apply his powers of observation to evaluate clues to the herbs' therapeutic powers, the remedial qualities, or the diseases for which these qualities are indicated. If at times the examples of correspondences throughout this work appear far-fetched, let me offer as warrants of the doctrine's usefulness some fifty-five years of living with and experiencing the healing herbs, as well as close to four decades of professional pharmacy and teaching of herbalism.

For the learner, the common or colloquial names of herbs

will often provide a close association with the remedy. There is a great deal more to such nomenclature than meets the unpracticed eye.

Plant names that refer to parts of the body include eyebright (*Euphrasia*), a specific for diseases of the eyes; liverwort (*Hepatica*), which has liver-like leaves and was used as a mild cleanser of that organ; mouthroot or gold thread, an excellent healer of mouth sores or ulcers. The leaves of heartsease (pansy) make a good cordial for the heart; kidneywort is a time-tested remedy for inflammation or stones of the kidney apparatus. Lung moss is healing in pulmonary complaints, and scullcap is still in demand as a nervine and antispasmodic.

Another group designates the specific applications of the herbs: cough herb, pukeweed, heal-all or self-heal, stoneseed, nosebleed, asthma weed, colic root, boneset, dysentery bark, feverwort, pilewort, scabwort, and so on.

The Indians had their own way of naming the plants. They indicated the use of the plant or particular part of the plant as shown above as "head" or "leg medicine," or described the appearance of the plant ("squirrel" or "beaver tail," or "thin" or "plump root"), or the taste ("sweet" or "bitter root"), or denoted the habitat ("swamp root") or origin ("Kickapoo remedy"). For example, the Ojibwes called the tamarack (*Larix laricina*) the "swamp tree," or *mucki-gwatig*, whose first name denotes the tree's parts as a cleanser of mucus—from the alimentary, kidney, and liver tracts. To all of this, the Indian medicine man added a suffix to the compound name indicating the part of the plant which is used, such as the flower or leaves. The Chippewas held to no exact terminology, and in naming the plants would often give the same name to several plants only because all served the same medicinal need. Many times one plant was given several names, each for a different use. Generally the names given by the Chippewas were compound nouns which indicated the appearance of the plant, the habitat, a peculiarity or characteristic of the plant, or its main use. The word often had a suffix, indicating the root, leaf, or flower, or other part of the plant to be utilized.

Each culture, each nation has had its own ways of assigning names to useful plants, and the Aztec Indians had theirs. Their medicinal plant names were often combined with the word *teo*, signifying "god" or "sacred." Examples are *teozquauitl* "sacred tree," *teoxihuitl* "sacred plant," *teoamatl* "sacred paper." And since these people felt that all matters of health and the healing of disease were decreed by their gods, they named many of their herb remedies after gods and goddesses: *totecyxiuh* (the herb of Totec, god of the goldsmiths), *capollaxipehuall* (black cherry of Xipe, goddess of flaying), *ayauhtl* (a plant named after Ayauh, the water goddess), *cozcanantzi* (jewel of Tonantzin, goddess of procreation).

By the same token, numerous herbs were named by Christians in past centuries in honor of Jesus and Mary and the saints. Christ's Eye is wild English clary (*Salvia verbenaca*), a folk remedy "to strengthen the eyesight," according to Culpepper. Christ's Thorn refers to the holly tree (*Ilex aquilofolium*), which, according to an old legend, sprang up wherever Christ trod the earth. Christ's Spear is none other than the English adder's tongue, which was considered a sovereign remedy for snake-bite. Christ's Ladder is centaury (*Erythraea centaurium*), which has ever been considered a quickly healing application for wounds. Marigold (*Calendula officinalis*) and Madonna Lily (*Convallaria majalis*) are dedicated to Mary; while Rosemary (*Rosemarinus officinalis*) was used by the ancients in Christmas decorations and in religious ceremonies, being highly revered by Europeans as one of the indigenous bushes that sheltered the Virgin Mary in the flight into Egypt. The Spanish call it *romero*, the Pilgrim's Flower. Writers of old applied the name St. Mary's Seal to the common Solomon's seal. And last, here are a few examples of plants named to honor Christian saints: St. John's Plant is the English mugwort, considered the herb with which John the Baptist girdled himself when in the wilderness. But St. John's Herb is agrimony (hemp) a name that has lasted since Bible days. The plant provided material for ropes which kept political prisoners bound to the stake. St. John's Bread is the edible carob or boxa, which tradition says was St. John's food in the desert wastelands. St. Johnswort refers, however, to the golden hypericum, whose leaves and flowers are employed as a fast-acting healer of wounds. St. James-wort is the common ragwort (*Senecio jacobaea*), of which the astringent and cooling leaves are still employed as a wash to inflamed areas, burns, and old sores. To the bulbous buttercup is given the name St. Anthony's Turnip and to the ubiquitous, weedy common hedge mustard is the name St. Barbara's Hedge Mustard given, which has the supposed property of remedying loss of voice.

Many animals have had plants named after them, for one association or another. Dog-Grass is the common witch grass which is sought out and eaten by small animals to induce vomiting. Horseheal is elecampane, a remedy for skin diseases of horses. Turtlehead refers only to the shape of the turtle's head but not to its uses, as does Cranesbill's seedpod to the bill of a crane. The Columbine was so named for its fancied resemblance to a circle of doves around a dish. Regarding Adder's Tongue, the generic name *Ophioglossum* is derived from *ophios*, "serpent," and *glossa*, "tongue," while the flower of the Snapdragon resembles the mouth of an animal. Cockscomb is the name given to yellow rattle, whose ripe, husky capsules cause a rattling of the seeds, its leaves resembling a cock's comb.

The signatures or hints given by certain characteristics of plants can be easily broken down into categories. Groups of plants sharing the same signature would probably be indicated for similar ailments or application to the same general area of the body. A variety of aspects of an individual plant can give us clues to its use : we should examine its habitat, its color, its shape, its texture, its odor, and its internal properties.

The first signature one might look for as an indication of an herb's specific therapeutic or healing property is its *habitat*.

Plants that grow in turgid brooks, wet lowlands, and swamps are associated with diseases of wetness : rheumatic disorders, feverish colds, and coughs. These plants include the willow, water pepper, mints, verbena, sweet flag, elder, boneset, jack-in-the-pulpit, and skunk cabbage.

Mucky soil signifies mucous excretions. When mucous excretions are excessive, an inflammation occurs along the membranes of the respiratory and genito-urinary passages which often develops into a diseased condition. The eucalyptus and sunflower are often cultivated in swampy areas to rid the places of foul, miasmatic conditions, and are similarly employed to cleanse out the "swampy" areas of the body.

Herbs and shrubs found growing on the banks of clear ponds and fast-moving brooks are mostly indicated as diuretics, such as horsetail, bedstraw, assorted aromatic mints, smartweed, black alder, water agrimony, and hydrangea. These plants can help to cleanse the urinary system of its waste and stone-forming deposits.

Herbs inhabiting gravelly places may also be found growing over large rock formations or completely covering sandy, barren areas. Such plants can help cleanse and remove from the mucous linings and from their associated areas—i.e. the alimentary and bronchial systems—the harmful stone-forming and catarrhal accumulations. An inflammation may be reduced and disease be prevented by the use of the following : bearberry, horsetail, peppergrass, parsley, parsley piert, shepherd's purse, juniper, may flower, gromwell, and the two "stone-breakers," sassafras and saxifrage.

The herb-studying novice should always remember that specimens of the same plant found in different locations will vary widely in the amounts of active medicinal ingredients each will yield. Milkweed growing in sandy soil will yield almost twice the active constituents as the same herb located in rich soil. There is also a vast difference between the potency of plants growing in the wild and the same plants which have been artificially cultivated or transferred from their original locations to soils readied by the hands of man. Transplanting and cultivation seem to cause unprofitable changes of their internal components. For example, the dandelion, usually small and concentrated when found in its natural locale, is effective in remedying afflictions of the liver and kidneys; but when it is artificially cultivated, starch sugar increases, as do other therapeutically useless ingredients.

The *color* of the plant's flower, fruit, or decoction from root or stem may also be a signature.

Those herbs with yellow flowers generally are indicated in disorders of the liver and gallbladder. It is the pathological symptom of the yellowness of a jaundice that provides the specific clue. Dandelion, jewel weed, wild snapdragon, hawkweed, tansy, and gentian are examples of this type of remedy.

Those plants with reddish flowers, such as red clover, burdock, rose, raspberry, bee balm, and pimpernel, have long been established as blood purifiers or alteratives, and may still be used as such today. A reddish color may also suggest the astringency or healing effect of a plant in external or skin disorders arising from blood impurities. (The active principles of many alterative plants are today considered "antibiotic.")

The same therapeutic actions are indicated for herbs with a similar yellow-orange or reddish hue presented by their fruits or by a decoction of their stems or roots. For instance, mandrake and lemon, with yellow-colored fruits, are considered useful remedies in jaundice and liver derangements. The reddish fruits of bearberry, mulberry, strawberry, hawthorn, and squaw vine indicate these herbs in diseases of the blood. A decoction of goldenseal, barberry, or gold thread yields a golden yellow color, on account of which this trio has enjoyed a well-deserved reputation in remedies for a troublesome or infected liver and gallbladder.

Plants with purple or blue flowers have been considered good for improving the complexion or the color of the skin. Joe-pye, red clover, verbena, burdock, gentian, and chicory are good examples and, though generally categorized as blood purifiers, are also suitable remedies for a pathological condition known as cyanosis. This is a blueness or purplish lividness of the skin's surface arising from a deficient oxygenation (respiratory-blood malfunction) which causes an impaired arterial flow of the bloodstream.

The *form* of the plant can also provide clues to its uses.

The pattern of growth taken by vines associates them with conditions of the nervous and blood systems, which of course take a similar form within the body. We can find the word "vine" in "vein," another mnemonic device. These herbs have been much employed as alteratives (blood purifiers) and as nervines or antispasmodics: sarsaparilla, American ivy (woodbine), licorice, bittersweet, grape, hops, cat-ivy and mints. The especially crawling growth of septfoil and cinquefoil indicates its "needle-and-thread" healing properties in skin conditions, while the very long, slender root (rhizome) of dog-grass and the trailing stems of the procumbent bearberry also specify use in blood disorders.

Parasitical growths like beech drops have a "sticking to" property. This herb was much used in a variety of skin disorders, thus earning its common synonym, cancer root.

Different *textures* indicate different uses.

Adhesiveness. A ground herb that clings to itself will cling to and remove the hardening mucus or irritating catarrh of the inner systems. Outstanding examples are sage, coltsfoot, hoarhound, everlasting, and mallow.

Plants whose leaves are soft in texture are to be used to ease the pain of a diseased or painful area. Mallow, malva species, hoarhound, hollyhock, and mullein are examples. No herb mixture intended for internal use is ever complete or satisfactory without one such emollient ingredient. The downy leaves of mullein, hoarhound, hollyhock, and woundwort were once used as a lint substitute for dressing wounds.

Those herbs with sharp thorns or prickles signify their application in cases of pain. The herbs are not anodynes or pain-relievers, but they are a most suitable means to strike at the causes of the pain. Hawthorn performs a dual function, acting as a diuretic and as a tonic for the heart. Stramonium, an antispasmodic and relaxant in bronchial spasms of asthma, is better known as an anodyne and narcotic, with properties similar to those of hyoscyamus and belladonna. Prickly lettuce is a pain reliever and sedative in coughs. Motherwort is especially indicated as an antispasmodic and nervine in female disorders and amenorrhea. Thistle is a stimulating tonic to the inner organs, helping greatly to relieve the pain and affliction of diseased liver and spleen. Raspberry, strawberry, and blackberry, by virtue of their acid constituents (malic and citric), act upon the tartar formations that lead to kidney and gallstones, thus relieving pain and discomfort.

The epidermal hairs (trichomes) of plants such as nettles, sumac, mullein, currant, primula, hops, and sundew suggest the use of these hairy herbs in various painful internal disorders, especially for conditions known as "a stitch in the side" or "pins-and-needles." Of the latter two herbs, hops is credited with calmative and anodyne properties whereas sundew, whose most sensitive hairs catch all insects which alight on them, has served well to stop the hurtful irritation and suffering caused by whooping cough or chronic bronchitis.

Skin-healers are indicated in various ways. The signature of the following herbs is their thin, thread-like stems and roots, suggesting the sewing up of skin lesions: bedstraw, cleavers, septfoil, cinquefoil, and gold thread. (Spider webs are also considered useful for this purpose.) Lenticels (openings in the

outer layer of cork and tissues of stems) also represent skin
lesions. White birch, elder, cherry, and sumac are indicated.

The spotted leaves of St. Johnswort are employed in the healing of tumorous spots or sores of the body. The wart-like excrescences of sumac and the inch-long galls of various oak trees
contain large amounts of tannic and gallic acids, which possess
astringent and healing properties. Balsamic and resinous exudations help to heal most lesions, cuts, and ulcers of the skin. They
include the balsams of peru, benzoin, storax, and tolu; the
resins of guaiac, mastic, pine, myrrh, cambogia, and turpentine;
and the dried juices of aloe and kino. Finally, lichens and molds
are useful in skin diseases such as psoriasis, which they resemble.

Further exudations may be of two kinds. A soft mucilaginous
texture may be obtained directly from the exudations of trees
or shrubs such as acacia and tragacanth. When dissolved in
water, this hardened substance swells to form an adhesive jelly
or mucilage. Or there is the thick, viscid liquid which is produced
by any of the following herbs when infused in hot water: Irish
moss, hollyhock, mallow species, lungwort, elm, and flaxseed.
In the former case, the resultant semi-liquid becomes a base for
oil preparation (e.g. acacia) and for the suspension of water-
insoluble chemical drugs and the manufacture of troches (throat
tablets). In the latter case, each herb is an active ingredient of
the entire herb mixture or preparation.

Aroma is another important signature. The ancients believed
that strong-smelling plants would drive away evil spirits and
so employed these aromatics as fumigants: cinnamon, clove,
arbor vitae, frankincense. Many pleasant-smelling herbs such
as thyme, rosemary, and juniper are still employed as disinfec-
tants and deodorizers, and are the herbs included in the *incensier* method of disinfecting rooms employed even today in
French hospitals. Aromatics such as marjoram, mint, rosemary,
and anise were employed in Elizabethan days to counteract
mouth odors, halitosis, and body odors. The active principles

of most aromatic herbs are highly antiseptic or germicidal and contain valuable antibiotic principles. Included in this category are the aforementioned herbs plus tansy, pennyroyal, sage, savory, fennel, and other food-seasoning herbs.

Several herbs have signatures which relate to features of the human body.

The hair of the head was represented by the hairs of the globular, head-shaped fruits of castor and burdock, both of which are used in hair preparations, while the shape of the head itself had its likeness in scullcap and walnut. The brain was represented by the walnut and by the fine-meshed root systems of valerian and lady's slipper which were said to resemble the brain structure. The latter two herbs have been much employed in nervous disorders, headaches, and the like.

The tubelike bronchial apparatus is represented by tubular foods like the green tops of onion, garlic, and others of that family. That organ also has its resemblance in the appearance of adult growth of thyme and Irish moss, herbs that are much employed in cough remedies.

The compact flower clusters of sumac, self-heal, and hard-hack indicate an accumulation of pus sacs in the throat or tonsils and are often employed by the commercial herbalist and in folk medicine as an astringent gargle for tonsillitis and sore throats. The peculiarly shaped corolla of throatwort appeared to the early herbalists as a most reasonable facsimile of that part of the body, and they found it of good service in the treatment of throat irritations.

Eyebright and chamomile have for centuries been used as lay remedies for diseases of the eyes, because of the claim that the herbs' floral parts resembled the eyes. Plants like mandragora, poke, ginseng, and bryony, whose root formations resemble the forked structure of the human groin, led the ancients to employ them as aphrodisiacs or as a means to overcome sterility.

One could go on and on listing examples of correspondences

between plant features and the use of that plant for human ailments. Remember that there are useful plants which do not have
a signature, and that not every signature is applicable in every
case. However, I believe that every plant, every tree, every
blade of grass has some virtue, perhaps still undiscovered, and
the signature theory in general has proven to be a most effective
way of teaching and learning those we know.

II

*An Herbal
of
Medicinal
Plants*

Plants from many parts of the Western Hemisphere are represented in this herbal, but most are common to the northern half of the United States and the southern part of Canada.

COLLECTION, DRYING, AND PRESERVATION OF THE HERBS

In general, the term "herb" refers to the overground portion of the plant, sometimes mentioned in the text as the "entire" herb or plant. The herb is gathered when in flower. However, it is advisable to gather and use only the upper half of the plant.

The *leaves:* Collect the whole plant or leaf-bearing stems when the plant is in flower and only on the *second* consecutive rainless day. Gather only those free from dew. Dry by suspension, strip the leaves from their stems, and store the leaves. Keep only those which have retained their full green color. While the large woody stems yield little medicinal virtue, they should be chopped up and placed in a compost pile or directly in the vegetable patch.

The *flowers:* Collect them just as they begin to open, and when they are free from dew. Spread to dry on a frame. Turn or shake them occasionally or daily to insure complete drying throughout and preservation of their natural color.

The *seeds:* They are gathered when nearly but not fully ripe, and before the seed pods or capsules have opened. Proceed as indicated under flowers.

The *bark and root:* These are generally gathered in the fall (though some writers suggest spring collections), or during the end of the herb's growing season. The outer rough bark is first scraped off before peeling and then the inner bark is removed. Roots that are collected during the course of the growing season often shrink excessively in the drying process and thus do not have optimum value. There are a few exceptions to the rule: the root of yellow dock may be gathered soon after "rusting" of the seed heads (in New England, during the last week of

July), and the roots of wild ginger, skunk cabbage, and jack-in-the-pulpit are gathered in the spring.

When you collect nettles or smartweed, be sure to wear gloves.

Directly after gathering fresh elder flowers and placing them in your car, be sure to keep the windows open. This herb must be dried in the attic or away from any area used for sitting or eating, because the volatile gaseous oil liberated from the flowers by sun or immediate warmth may cause dizziness or headache.

Freshly-gathered aromatics, such as catnip, mints, or chamomile, must be spread loosely and quickly dried by suspension, and not be kept bunched together too long directly after collection, in order to prevent the possibility of mold formation.

To dry whole herbs (also leaves or flowers), suspend them, with the stems up and tied with string, near to the ceiling of a warm and well air-circulated room, attic, or cellar.

Do not crowd the material.

Keep the herb bunches away from the direct sunlight or indirect rays, to better preserve their natural appearance and optimum value.

The degree of "fragrance retention" of garden-grown aromatic seasonings (basil, marjoram, balm, etc.), their leaves and seeds, depends upon proper harvesting and drying procedures. They are gathered in the morning after the dew has dried on them and before the sun becomes too warm. Such plants are harvested when the plants come into bloom, for then they contain the highest amount of essential aromatic oil. Small bunches of the herbs are tied together and hung upside down on a stretched line to dry. A small space is allowed between bunches to permit air to pass through them. Leaves, flowers, and seeds may be dried on an elevated drying frame (such as a converted window screen). Circulation of air is enhanced by placing the screen frames across blocks or in any position where air can reach the underside as well as the top of each frame, and by having a small electric fan nearby, directed away from the frame to avoid blowing the herbal plants.

The roots must be washed well before being set out to dry. They are either brush-scrubbed or placed on a wire mesh frame and briskly sprayed with a garden hose. The excess water dried off, the roots are sliced lengthwise or crosswise and spread in thin layers on a wooden attic floor, on screening or wire trays, or on flat metal containers situated on a warm oil burner. A daily shake of the herbs or container is necessary, as is protection from humidity. It is important that the roots are dried quickly at a warm temperature, but not one too high to injure the active ingredients. Exceptions to this rule are mayweed (fetid chamomile), which should be dried at least one month before using, skunk cabbage roots, one week, and jack-in-the-pulpit two to three weeks.

Once the herbs are identified, collected, and dried, one has a fresh source of herbs whose parts are stored as is and reduced in size only when needed. The label of every container of herbs should state the name of the herb, date of collection, and original location of the herb.

To be therapeutically active, the herbs or herb parts must be properly protected not only against the ever-present dangers of mold and uneven temperatures, since in the presence of warmth and moisture mold spores germinate very quickly, but moreover, against the ever-present threat of attack by moths and the tiny beetle, *Sitodrepa panicea*. As a general rule, the leaves or upper portion of a non-aromatic herb, after being well dried and finely ground, are best kept in wide-mouthed glass jars or cardboard boxes. However, all fleshy roots, such as the aforementioned burdock, must be preserved in airtight containers, glass or tin, that have been thoroughly washed with hot water and soap and dried. Some chemical preservative is then added: carbon tetrachloride or chloroform, paradichlorbenzene, camphor, or naphthalene moth crystals. A few drops of either liquid are applied to a two-inch square of thick absorbent cotton and placed between two sheets of waxed paper large enough to cover the width of the container; or a few large crystals of the solid preservative, wrapped in either cotton or paper, are placed both below and above the herbs. Seeds and flowers of aromatic herbs need no such care.

Store all herbs in a cool place.

Duration of the herbs' value varies. Entire herbs and leaves may be kept two years, flowers and fruits two to three years, and roots three to four years, except for burdock, dandelion, poke, and other fleshy roots, which should be replaced every year.

ACACIA
Acacia senegal

SYNONYM   Gum Arabic

PART USED   Dried, gummy exudation. The gum of the acacia exudes spontaneously from cracks in the bark and hardens on exposure; in commercial production incisions are usually made in order to facilitate the exudation.

SIGNATURE   The exudation of the gum yielded by the tree bark.

SPECIFIC USE   Gum arabic is recorded by Herodotus as being used by the ancient Egyptians as an adhesive. Its use in medicine is mentioned in several of the Egyptian papyri. Hippocrates refers to it in medical works published between 450 and 350 B.C.

The viscidity of a solution of the gum of acacia indicates its value in removing phlegm from the throat and bronchia. Such a solution is demulcent in action, serving to reduce inflammatory conditions of the respiratory and digestive organs. Alone, the gum, because of its glutinous quality, exerts a soothing influence upon irritated mucous tissue in the throat.

AGRIMONY
Agrimonia eupatoria

PARTS USED   The overground herb. The small yellow flowers, which are borne on slender terminal spikes.

SIGNATURE   The whole plant yields a yellow color.

SPECIFIC USE   Yellowing of the eyes was diagnosed by the early Greek physicians, as by modern physicians, as symptomatic of a liver disorder. The herb is an effective remedy for jaundice and liver complaints. The leaves and the small yellow flowers emit a most pleasing apricot-like aroma for which purpose the herb is much used by Europeans as a refreshing tea.

WATER AGRIMONY
Bidens tripartita

SYNONYM   Bur Marigold

SIGNATURE   This is an annual plant which is found in wet places, on the borders of ponds or ditches. Its composite flower heads are brownish yellow.

SPECIFIC USE   The herb has been employed in kidney disorders and liver troubles.

BLACK ALDER
Prinos verticillatus

SYNONYM   Winterberry, Feverbush

PARTS USED   Fruits, bark.

SIGNATURE   1. The fruits are a bright scarlet.
    2. The outer dark brown surface is spotted with whitish patches and black dots and lines.
    3. The inner bark is yellow and imparts a yellow-saffron color to the saliva.

4. This shrub is found in moist woods and on the banks of swamps and brooks.

SPECIFIC USE 1. Black alder bark is widely used in blood disorders, indolent sores, and chronic skin ailments. For this purpose, it is often combined with burdock, yellow dock, and sarsaparilla.

2. Ulcerated skin lesions and skin diseases are here indicated. A suitable preparation of the ground bark may be obtained by simmering in unsalted lard or vegetable oil, or allowing to soak in alcohol for eight to ten days.

3. Signatures 3 and 4 relate to the herb's use in liver and gallbladder derangements, especially where jaundice or dyspepsia is indicated. It helps to cleanse the system of accumulated mucoid toxins.

TAG ALDER
Alnus serrulata

PARTS USED The bark and cones.

SIGNATURE 1. The small corky warts on the bark.

2. It grows in wetness, on the borders of swamps and ponds.

SPECIFIC USE 1. A strong decoction of the bark and cones yields astringent-healing properties useful for various skin diseases.

2. The parts have been much used as a diuretic and alterative in kidney and rheumatic disorders.

ALKANET
Alkanna tinctoria

SYNONYMS Dyer's Bugloss, Dyer's Anchusa (not to be confused with the true Anchusa or Bugloss, *Anchusa officinalis*)

SIGNATURE The yellow to purplish-blue corolla and the red dye of the root.

SPECIFIC USE   It is indicated in diseases of the organs associated with the bloodstream—those of the liver, spleen, and gallbladder.

WILD ALLSPICE
Lindera benzoin

SYNONYM   Benjamin Bush

PARTS USED   Fruits, leaves, twigs.

SIGNATURE   The habitat is one of wetness: swamps and wet soil.

SPECIFIC USE   Herbalists have long recommended its use as a febrifuge. It is suggested that wild allspice be mixed half and half with other herbs. During the War of Independence the spicy berries were used by the Americans as a substitute for imported allspice, and the leaves as a tea substitute. Later, and for some 100 years, all the parts came to be employed as a fever-breaker in colds.

ALOE
(Socrotine Aloe, *Aloe perryi,* Curacao or Bitter Aloe, *A. barbadensis,* Cape Aloe, *A. ferox*)

PART USED   The dried juice of the leaves.

SIGNATURE   The thick yellow juice that exudes from the fleshy leaf when cut.

SPECIFIC USE   The juice, dried or fresh, has long been used externally for all types of skin disorders. For chapped or rough hands and insect bites, the *freshly expressed juice* is applied directly, and similarly in the case of sunburn or scald. For the latter conditions, a strong warm decoction of pekoe tea is prepared, to which Irish moss is added to form a jelly. To this mixture the clear gummy juice of the aloe is added. This preparation has been found to be most soothing and healing. The dried aloe juice is an ingredient of Compound Tincture of Benzoin which is today employed for its antiseptic and protective effect as a local application to minor wounds, indolent ulcers, and so forth.

AMARANTH
Amaranthus hypochondriacus

The name is from the Greek word meaning "unwithering," and was applied to those plants which seemingly lasted forever, thus signifying immortality.

SYNONYMS   Garden or Red Amaranth, Velvet Flower

PARTS USED   Flowers, leaves, and root.

SIGNATURE   The spike-borne, velvety, purple to blood-red flowers.

SPECIFIC USE   Herbalist Culpepper recommended the flowers as an aid to "stop all fluxes of blood, whether in man or woman, bleeding in the nose or wound." The modern herbalist will similarly use the flowers, leaves, and root as a healing astringent for external ulcers and sores, for mouth ulcers, for hemorrhage of the bowels, and in bleeding piles. Because of their antiseptic-astringent properties, a strong decoction of this and the wild amaranth is often used as a gargle and wash for mouth sore, cankers, and bleeding and ulcerated gums.

ANGELICA
A. atropurpurea

PARTS USED   The leaves, seeds, and roots.

SIGNATURE   1. The stems are hollow.
    2. The plant grows in areas of wetness, in damp soil.

SPECIFIC USE   1. Angelica has been much used, by virtue of its medicinal and aromatic properties, to loosen and eliminate the catarrhal discharges from the alimentary, bronchial, and urinary systems.

2. The herb is a stimulating diaphoretic and expectorant for colds, coughs, and pleurisy. It is also a good remedy for rheumatism and kidney disorders. The herb's property of carminative and stomachic serves well in colic and flatulence.

APPLE
Pyrus malus

PART USED   The whole fruit.

SIGNATURE   1. The red color.
  2. The seeds.

SPECIFIC USE   1. While not a true blood purifier, the apple will certainly enrich the blood. It will, states one authority, "often reduce acidity of the stomach, and corrects sour fermentation." One might say that the sugar of sweet apples, like most fruit sugars, may be considered a "predigested food" in that it quickly passes into and fortifies the bloodstream. The body is thus provided with extra energy and warmth. An apple is completely digested and assimilated in about one and a half hours. To obtain the optimum food value of this fruit, eat it unpeeled and uncooked, since the most valuable nutrients exist within and just beneath the skin.

The malic and tartaric acids, perhaps the apple's chief dietetic value, are a remedy for liver problems. These fruit acids also serve to neutralize the waste products of gout and rheumatism. Furthermore, unless waste products are removed from our bodies, the blood will suffer from these toxins. Cases of constipation and biliousness, however mild or severe, will be relieved by the eating of a ripe and juicy apple an hour or so before retiring, and again in the morning.

2. The seeds of all fruits such as apples, grapes, or plums represent kidney stones, i.e., the cumulative result of hardened gravel (and of faulty dietary habits) ; they also designate the fruit's ability to assist in eliminating stone from the body. The apple also serves as a dentifrice for it cleanses the teeth by removing the tartar deposits which are said to be the beginning of kidney stones.

ARBOR VITAE
Thuja occidentalis

SYNONYMS   Tree of Life, Hackmatack, "Yellow Cedar" (the true Yellow Cedar is *Juniperus virginiana*)

PART USED   The recently dried leafy twigs.

SIGNATURE   1. The small but conspicuous flattened oil glands found on the back of the twig-end leaves.

2. This large evergreen tree grows in low swampy areas and along streams. It is often grown as a hedge on home grounds.

3. The fresh dried leaf branches have a strongly pungent and balsamic odor.

SPECIFIC USES   1. It is much used in various skin diseases and as an application to warts and other excrescences. For this purpose, the leaves are made into an ointment or into an alcoholic tincture.

2. The leaves were recommended by European physicians of the 1800s for dropsy and general urinary disorders, but because of their abortifacient properties their use was discontinued. A warm infusion of the leaves is today used by some in colds and intermittent fevers, but the writer considers this inadvisable.

3. The generic name *Thuja* is taken from the Greek word meaning "to fumigate" or from *thuo*, "to sacrifice," the aro-

matic balsamic wood having been burned by the ancients at sacrifice altars. The arbor vitae presents us with a strong and quickly prepared disinfectant for sick-room needs, capable of eliminating foul odors and preventing the spread of contagious infections. A handful of this herb, plus one of tansy and juniper, stirred well in a quart of hot water, will almost immediately yield the needed antiseptic vapors.

TRAILING ARBUTUS
Epigoea repens

SYNONYMS   Mayflower, Gravel Plant, Ground Laurel

PARTS USED   The leaves. Also, the whole plant.

SIGNATURE   It is found principally in wet sandy woods or gravelly soil. The generic name *Epigoea* is a Greek word signifying "upon the ground," thus indicating its mode of growth and trailing habit.

SPECIFIC USE   Until recently, it was much used as a diuretic for all urinary disorders. It is especially good as an antilithic to remove stone and gravel (as its synonym suggests).

ARRACH
Chenephodium olidum

SYNONYMS   Stinking Arrach, Stinking Goosefoot, Stinking Motherwort

PART USED   The whole herb.

SIGNATURE   1. When the whitish, greasy mealiness that covers the herb is roughly handled or removed, it emits a lasting, rather foul odor—thus the synonyms.
    2. The mealy substance covering the entire plant.

SPECIFIC USE   1. A decoction of the herb was formerly employed as a wash for external ulcers or sores yielding an objectionable odor.

2. Similarly, the nervous system covers the entire body, thus signifying the herb's nervine and antispasmodic properties. It is used to some extent in nervous disorders, hysteria and "female complaints" (thus the synonym Motherwort).

ARROWHEAD
Sagittaria latifolia

SYNONYMS Tule Potato, Wapatoo

PART USED The corms (tubers).

SIGNATURE The plant is a constant resident of wet areas and shallow ponds.

SPECIFIC USE Diuretic.

JERUSALEM ARTICHOKE
Helianthus tuberosus

This plant is not a native of Jerusalem or of the Near East, as the name implies. "Jerusalem" is a corruption of the Italian *girasola*, "turning to the sun."

SYNONYM Sunflower Artichoke

PART USED The tubers.

SIGNATURE These tuberous sunflowers claim their habitat along the banks of brooks and in wet places.

SPECIFIC USE In common with other sunflowers, the leaves of the Jerusalem artichoke have long been used by the peoples of Europe in the treatment of malarial fever. A tincture of the flowers has been recommended in the treatment of bronchiectasis.

ASPARAGUS
Asparagus officinalis

PARTS USED   The edible shoots. The roots.

SIGNATURE   It is found growing wild along seacoasts and in moist waste areas. The new shoots are very juicy and succulent, containing 94% water.

SPECIFIC USE   This is the well-known table vegetable. Used as a table dish, asparagus stimulates the kidneys. All parts, but especially the new shoots, possess strong diuretic properties. The active ingredient, asparagine, has been employed in cardiac dropsy, the fluid extract in chronic nephritis. The root has been found most helpful in removing gravel from the urinary system. A warm tea of the herb may be taken at three-to-four-hour intervals to promote a free flow of urine. One health author informs us that the expressed juice serves well in rheumatism, since it helps to break up the oxalic acid crystals in the kidneys and throughout the muscular system.

BALM OF GILEAD
Poplar Buds, *Populus candicans,* Tacamahac or Balsam Poplar, *P. tacamahaca*

PART USED   Closed buds, collected in late winter.

SIGNATURE   The resinous exudation covering the scaled leaf-buds.

SPECIFIC USE   As a vulnerary, the buds are simmered in lard to prepare an ointment or placed in alcohol to prepare a tincture, both of which are intended to heal skin eruptions, scratches, bruises, or swellings. The buds are considered a stimulating expectorant in bronchial disorders and therefore employed as an ingredient of various cough syrups.

FIR BALSAM
Abies balsamea

SYNONYMS   American Silver Fir, Balsam Tree, Canada Balsam

PART USED   The oleoresinous exudation.

SIGNATURE   The resinous exudations which form naturally upon the blistered bark of the trunk and branches.

SPECIFIC USE   See Balm of Gilead.

BARBERRY
Berberis vulgaris

SYNONYMS   Sourberry, Berbery

PARTS USED   Although the bark of the root is "officially"* indicated, the whole root, the fruits, and the stem are also used.

SIGNATURE   1. All inner parts, and especially the roots, of this bushy herb declare a yellow color which is much sought as a dye.
2. The red, football-shaped fruits.
3. The thorns.

SPECIFIC USE   1. It is of excellent service as a hepatic and stimulating tonic in jaundice, dyspepsia, and the usual gallbladder and liver disorders.
2. The mature fruits are juiceless but highly acidulous and antiscorbutic, and serve well to protect the bloodstream from metabolic wastes. From the fruits, a jam, jelly, or preserve may be prepared.
3. The sharp thorns signify pain; thus the herb is used when pain accompanies disorders of the liver and gallbladder.

---

* As recognized in the *United States Pharmacopoeia* and the *National Formulary* or in similar medical compendia.

KIDNEY BEAN
Phaseolus vulgaris

SYNONYM   French Bean

PART USED   The seeds.

SIGNATURE   The spotted seeds are kidney-shaped.

SPECIFIC USE   In the mid-eighteenth century, they were found to be a most wholesome food, and, together with their young pods, were considered to be of a diuretic nature and to cleanse the kidneys and ureters of gravel.

BEARBERRY
Arctostaphylos uva-ursi

SYNONYMS   Mountain Box, Rockberry, Uva Ursi, Upland Cranberry

PARTS USED   The dried evergreen leaves. The fruits.

SIGNATURE   The thick masses of the herb are found growing only over large rocky areas and extremely sandy, gravelly places. Also the red berries, containing five one-seeded stones.

SPECIFIC USE   This herb offers an original example of the doctrine of signatures. A microscopic examination of a cross-section of the leaf reveals, equidistant from the center of the leaf (representing the human spinal cord) two masses of kidney-shaped, thick-walled cells. Possessing diuretic-antiseptic properties, the leaves have indeed been found useful in chronic kidney disorders, cystitis, and catarrh of the urinary organs. Used with leaves, the fruits are considered antilithic, in that they help to dissolve and eliminate stone and gravel from the kidney apparatus. In either case both an aromatic and a demulcent must be added to a preparation of the leaves or berries, since their action when taken alone is too strong and irritating. The herb's use was well known to the North American Indians.

BEE BALM
Monarda didyma

SYNONYMS   Bergamot, Oswego Tea, Red Monarda

PART USED   The whole herb.

SIGNATURE   1. The pale green leaflets appear in pairs along the square stem.
2. The plant prefers a somewhat moist soil.
3. The showy flowers are of a brilliant scarlet color.
4. Its strong but pleasant aroma.

SPECIFIC USE   The first two signatures place this herb in the category of kidney stimulants. The third one reminds us that it serves to remove impurities from the bloodstream and to stimulate the liver and spleen, containing, as it does, a high percentage of thymol, a powerful antiseptic. As for the last signature, the herb is much used as an aromatic bitter for nervous stomach. The blossoms of bee balm and of many other aromatic herbs secrete much nectar and so become favorites of the bees, but it must be remembered that the leaves of these plants, in turn, become antidotes for bee and other insect stings.

BEECH
Fagus americana

SYNONYM   Beechnut Tree

PARTS USED   The leaves and nuts.

SIGNATURE   The recurved spines of the nut burs.

SPECIFIC USE   As a child I collected vast amounts of the leafy twigs for my grandfather's kidney remedies. But it was not until I discovered the reason for such an employment that I came to understand its signature. The Indians called this the water beech and used it for pains in the lower back but its habitat is generally not one of wetness. John Gerard (1597) noted

the connection: water is found in the tree's "hollownesse."
Spiny burs indicated pain, or better, the relief of pain, and the
kernels, stated Gerard, "are reported to ease the paine of the
kidnies if they be eaten."

BEECH DROPS
Epifagus virginiana

SYNONYMS   Broom Rape, Cancer Root

SIGNATURE   The parasitical type of growth formed on beech
tree roots indicates its healing ("sticking to") property. The
dull red color of the freshly collected drops suggests a poor
bloodstream.

SPECIFIC USE   A strong, cooled decoction was, and still is, applied as an external application in skin disorders, ulcers, and
erysipelas, and is said to arrest gangrene. The *U.S. Dispensatory* tells us that the herb was called cancer root because of its
folk use as a local application to cancerous ulcers.

As to its internal application, its use is indicated for its
astringent-healing properties. The decoction (one part to
three parts warm water) has been employed as a quickly binding action in diarrhea. But more important, we note that despite its slightly nauseous bitter taste, teas of the herb have
been taken for bleeding internal ulcers with astonishingly lasting results.

RED BEET
Beta vulgaris

SIGNATURE   The red color. The name *Beta* is derived from
the Celtic word meaning "red."

SPECIFIC USE   The beet enriches the bloodstream. One may
consume this excellent food in one of several ways: as the
grated vegetable, as a freshly prepared juice, or as a recently

blenderized product. If the food must be heated, steam it for a few minutes in as little water as possible, *without removing the skin*. Thus the blood-fortifying minerals are preserved. Furthermore, one should eat the greens as near raw as possible, for they, too, are an important article of food. Contained in the beet are these essential minerals: calcium, chlorine, potassium, silicon, sodium, and sulfur. Only by eating the beet uncooked is it possible to retain all the minerals, *and in proper balance*. The beet therapy, for whatever its healing or blood enriching purpose, must be carried on for at least six to eight weeks to show the required improvement.

COMMON BIRCH
Betula alba

SYNONYM   White Birch

PARTS USED   The vernal sap. The bark and its oil. The leaves.

SIGNATURE   When the tree's bark is wounded, the saccharine sap oozes out. Yellow fungous excrescences swell out from the fissures of the wood. Also, the bark and twigs are covered with numerous horizontally elongated lenticels. These signatures foretell their uses in external skin disorders.

SPECIFIC USE   The white outer layer of the bark has often been employed to yield the oil of birch tar, while the bark itself contains a fair amount of tannic acid. The mildly astringent but fast-healing oil has been extensively utilized as a parasiticide and antiseptic in skin affections such as eczema; a large decoction of the bark and leaves was used to bathe similar skin eruptions. The swelling wood excrescences were used by American and Canadian Indians as a moxa for warts.

BLACKBERRY
Rubus species

SYNONYM   Bramble, Goutberry, Dewberry

PARTS USED   Leaves, fruits, and roots.

SIGNATURE   1. The thorns.
2. The many-seeded fruit.

SPECIFIC USE   1. The thorns indicate painful symptoms arising from and associated with the organic disorders herein noted,
and certainly do not indicate any special anodyne properties.
Rather do these sharp prickles point to the herb's therapeutics
which may help the herb user to overcome his ailment.

2. Such seeded fruits have for centuries been employed to
dissolve out dangerous tartarous matter, starting with the tartar deposited upon the teeth by wrong diet. The ripe fruits are
juicy and pleasantly flavored and should be eaten in large quantities when in season. It is the citric and malic acids of the fruit
that help to counteract and dissolve tartar deposits in the
mouth, along the alimentary system, and in the areas of the kidney and gallbladder. (See also Barberry, Raspberry, Strawberry.)

The unripe fruits and the fall-collected roots are well known
for their tannic acid content which renders these parts an effective astringent for dysentery and diarrhea, as well as a gargle
for thrush and other irritations of the throat.

BLACK-EYED SUSAN
Rudbeckia hirta

SYNONYM   Yellow Coneflower

PART USED   The root system.

SIGNATURE   The high cone, composed of purplish brown
florets.

SPECIFIC USE   The cone clearly resembles the shape of a suppurating boil, and thus the herb has been advantageously employed by herbalists in the usual blood and skin diseases. Today scientific researchers have shown that its extracts possess effective antibiotic action against the *Staphylococcus aureus* bacteria. Garden rudbeckia (purple coneflower), a close relative of the above herb, was at one time considered by the physician an effective alterative in blood disorders, and in the treatment of septicemia, boils, and indolent ulcers. The *U.S. Dispensatory* attributes to coneflowers the distinct property of increasing the body's resistance to infection.

BLOODROOT
Sanguinaria canadensis

The Indians used the red juice of the root to decorate their bodies, clothes, and weapons, but do not apply the fresh juice to your own skin for you may be as sensitive to it as to poison ivy. Most tribes valued the herb also as a remedy for numerous ailments, of which some are here mentioned.

SYNONYMS   Red Puccoon, Tetterwort, Indian Red Paint

PART USED   The root system.

SIGNATURE   1. The habitat—mucky soil of rich woods.
2. The red coloring matter.

SPECIFIC USE   1. It has been much used as a stimulating expectorant and as an aid to remove the mucous accumulations from the bronchial tubes in bronchitis and asthmatic complaints.
2. Bloodroot is recorded as an invaluable alterative for impure conditions of the blood and torpidity of the liver. The slow exudation of the red blood-like juice from the broken fleshy root-stalk also taught the Indian medicine man to use a decoc-

tion of the herb as an application to fungous growths, open ulcers, and fleshy excrescences. Cherokee medicine men, also observing the herb's red juice oozing out like blood, recommended a decoction of this and three other native herbs to be drunk by women to promote menstruation.

BONESET
Eupatorium perfoliatum

SYNONYMS   Ague Weed, Indian Sage, Thoroughwort

PART USED   The upper half of the plant.

SIGNATURE   1. The herb is found in moist lowlands, in swamps, and along the banks of brooks and streams.

2. The bases of the two lance-shaped leaves are united, giving the appearance of the stalk piercing the center of one long leaf, as the specific name, *perfoliatum,* suggests.

SPECIFIC USE   1. Because of its habitat, it was much used by the Indians and early colonists as a diaphoretic, tonic, and febrifuge in diseases of wetness—systemic colds, influenza, fevers, and bronchial disorders. It is generally combined with all laxative and anti-dyspepsia herbs, as its catarrh removal action helps to improve the condition of the mucous membranes of the alimentary and bronchial systems, the bowels, and the liver. Because of this signature and its cleansing effect upon almost all of the body's organs, it was considered a near "cureall" and was included in almost all herb remedies.

2. The Indian medicine man, noting how the two leaves are joined together as if to indicate a fusion of broken leaves, used the plant in healing broken bones. Indeed, it is much recommended as a "rejuvenating tonic" for broken health. But the name Boneset is derived from its unquestioned value in treatment of breakbone fever. Recent herbal literature also declares the worth of this herb in the treatment of muscular rheumatism.

AMERICAN BROOKLIME
Veronica officinalis

EUROPEAN BROOKLIME
Veronica beccabunga

We have gathered much of this brightly blue-eyed brooklime as a most desirable substitute for the now uncommon water-cress. Not one of the *Veronica* species is poisonous, though eating its fresh leaves reminds one of watercress's pungency. The specific name *beccabunga* is from the Flemish *beckpunge,* "mouth smart," a synonym much used by Europeans.

SYNONYMS   Speedwell, Water Pimpernel (Water Speedwell, *Veronica anagallis-aquatica*)

PART USED   The entire herb.

SIGNATURE   1. All species are found in wet places—near springs, at the sides of brooks and ditches, and in swampy areas.
2. The dense covering of hairs over the leaves.

SPECIFIC USE   1. Brooklime has decided diuretic and toxic-cleansing properties and is most useful in all urinary, skin, and blood disorders. It is a recognized solvent-eliminator of the harmful gravel and stone from the kidneys as well as catarrhal deposits along the alimentary and bronchial canals.
2. The hairs represent the tickling sensation of a temporary throat irritation. The herb has been employed to remove the hardening mucus in coughs, bronchitis, and asthmatic conditions.

BROOM
Cytisus scoparius

PART USED   The early tops of the flowering branches.

SIGNATURE   The plants grow in sandy, stony soil, near streams of water.

SPECIFIC USE   It was employed principally as a specific for dropsy, its action, when used alone, being at the same time both diuretic and laxative. But when used with bearberry and dandelion root, broom tops have been found useful in cleansing the gravel from the urinary organs.

BUCKBEAN
Menyanthes trifoliata

SYNONYMS   Bogbean, Marsh Trefoil, Water Shamrock

PARTS USED   The leaves and roots.

SIGNATURE   1. The yellow (edible) fruit.
2. The mucky bogs and marshes in which the herb grows.

SPECIFIC USE   1. The yellow color of the fruit indicates its value as a remedy in jaundice and liver complaints.

2. Because it helps to remove mucous accumulations from the system, it serves as a deobstruent to remove the resultant gas and excessive acid, and therefore is most useful in dyspepsia, skin diseases, and gouty rheumatism.

BUGLEWEED
Lycopus virginicus

SYNONYMS   Gypsyweed, Pasture or Meadow Bugle

PART USED   The herb.

SIGNATURE   1. The habitat is moist lowland.
2. The lower sides of the leaves are gland-dotted.

SPECIFIC USE   1. The herb has long been held in high repute to relieve throat irritations, to loosen the phlegm, and to alleviate accompanying pain caused by coughs and bronchial disorders.

2. Its astringent property makes it a valuable healing agent

both internally and externally. It is a most effective remedy for diarrhea and dysentery, where hemorrhage is indicated.

VIPER'S BUGLOSS
Echium vulgare

SYNONYM Blueweed

PART USED The herb.

SIGNATURE 1. The seeds resemble the head of a snake. Thus, the generic name is derived from *echis,* "viper."
2. It grows in gravel pits, quarries, and stony areas.

SPECIFIC USE 1. It was considered a most efficacious antidote for snakebite.
2. It has been long employed as a demulcent-diuretic in the removal of gravelly deposits from the kidney tract.

BURDOCK
Articum lappa

SYNONYMS Burs, Beggar's Buttons

PARTS USED The leaves, fruits, and roots. The leaf stalks of the fruit of the first year's growth.

SIGNATURE 1. The flower heads.
2. The seeds of the fruits.
3. The color of the leaf stalks.

SPECIFIC USE 1. Because the round flower head was said to resemble the human head, and the prickles to resemble the hair, the fruits were and still are included in herbal hair tonics. Similarly did the resemblance of the individual flower head and its flowers to a festering boil cause the roots and the burs to be sought after for their strongly depurative and alterative properties. For this purpose the herbalist has long recommended a root mixture of burdock, dandelion, sarsaparilla, and yellow dock.

2. The hard seeds enclosed in the globular fruits designate the herb's application in the removal of stone and gravel deposits from the urinary organs. And indeed the fruits are indicated in dropsical complaints and the roots in the usual kidney disorders.

3. The red color rising from the base to halfway up the stem denotes its time-honored employment as a blood purifier. As preventative medicine the stalks of the spring-to-early-summer collection should be considered a worthy vegetable. Stripped of their rinds and prepared like asparagus, they form a delicious vegetable, far more nutritious than much store-bought produce.

BUTTER AND EGGS
Antirrhinum linaria

SYNONYMS   Wild Snapdragon, Toadflax

PART USED   The herb.

SIGNATURE   1. The yellow flowers.
2. The habitat—dry, sandy soil.

SPECIFIC USE   1. For centuries this herb has been employed primarily as a hepatic laxative in disorders of the liver and spleen and for jaundice.

2. The habitat indicated its application as a diuretic-eliminant when combined with antilithics and other diuretics, to remove gravel formations along the urinary tract.

CABBAGE
Brassica species

PART USED   The head.

SIGNATURE   The cabbage, when cut horizontally, will appear as a spinal cord and a diaphragm- or chest-like area showing stem-clasping leaves.

SPECIFIC USE   Since the spinal cord has always represented the nervous system, cabbage was at one time employed as a specific for mental and nervous disorders, for which two of its major ingredients, calcium and sulfur, are similarly prescribed by present-day physicians. Thus, its former use was also as a remedy for insomnia.

The transverse cutting demonstrates the application of the signature to the human diaphragm. Its various therapeutic uses included its being prescribed in chest and stomach remedies. Earlier in the century, even the most eminent of English doctors highly recommended the "French Formula for Chest Ailment," a decoction of red cabbage in water to which an equal amount of honey was added. (The French generally referred to this remedy as the "English Remedy.") Recently an extract of cabbage has come into prominence in the treatment of internal ulcers. It is reported that a concentrate of the juice appears to speed the healing of peptic ulcers and to reduce painful symptoms quite soon after administration.

CARROT
Daucus carota

SYNONYM   Philtron

PART USED   The whole plant.

SIGNATURE   The deep orange color.

SPECIFIC USE   Before the discovery of the relationship of vitamin A to eye deficiencies, the root was considered a specific and excellent deobstruent in liver disorders and jaundice. There is often a direct association between a diseased liver and poor eyesight. Poor eyesight may mean a vitamin A deficiency which must be corrected by cleansing the liver of its toxins and restoring the required vitamin content.

An Herbal of Medicinal Plants

CASSIA
Cassia fistula

SYNONYMS   Cassia Fruit, Purging Cassia

PART USED   The dried fruit.

SIGNATURE   The fruit is a dark brown cylindrical loment, shaped like a human stool.

SPECIFIC USE   The medicine is easily obtained by boiling the crushed fruits and evaporating the strained liquid to a thick but soft consistency. The result is a concentrated extract of sugar, mucilage, and a laxating substance.

CASTOR
Ricinus communis

SYNONYMS   Castor Bean, Castor-Oil Plant, Palma Christi

SIGNATURE   The soft spines that cover the fruits.

SPECIFIC USE   The literature states that even some 4,000 years ago the plant was utilized by the Egyptians in several ways. The Papyrus of 1552 B.C. recommended the seeds as a laxative and hair tonic and the oil for boils and in ointments. The oil today is much used in hair lotions and ointments which are intended to heal irritations of the scalp.

CAT-IVY
Nepeta hederacea, N. glechoma

SYNONYMS   Ground Ivy, Robin-Run-Around, Gill-over-the-Ground

PART USED   The entire plant.

SIGNATURE   1. The opposite kidney-shaped leaves.
  2. The herb's habitat—damp, shady places.

3. The long vine-like trailing stems. Its popular name, Ground Ivy, and botanical name, *hederacea,* signify its ivy-like growth.

4. The hairy tumors and the gland-dotted undersides of the leaves.

SPECIFIC USE   1 & 2. It is much used today as a stimulating diuretic in all urinary disorders.

3. Culpepper advised that to speedily heal external ulcers and fresh sores one should add a little honey to a decoction of cat-ivy, which then is "bound thereto."

4. A combination of the herb with yarrow and/or chamomile makes an excellent poultice for boils, tumors, and abscesses.

CATNIP
Nepeta cataria

PARTS USED   The leaves and flowering tops.

SIGNATURE   Its mint-like aromatic principles.

SPECIFIC USE   A most useful stimulating carminative and alkalizer-antacid in halitosis caused by stomach distress, and in colic and flatulence.

CELANDINE
Chelidonium majus

SYNONYMS   Tetterwort, Swallow-wort

PART USED   The entire herb.

SIGNATURE   The yellow flowers and the orange-colored juice.

SPECIFIC USE   From such writers as Dioscorides, Galen, and Forestus, one learns that the herb served as a most effectual remedy for the following situations: its diuretic-laxative property is noted, as it was during and since the days of Pliny, in cases of jaundice and in disorders of the liver and gallbladder. One of its ingredients, berberine, is the active principle of barberry (see above).

The fresh, slowly exuding orange juice indicates its property of healing ringworm (therefore the synonym Tetterwort), warts, corns, and other excrescences. Internally it was recommended for eczema and scrofulous diseases.

CELERY
Apium graveolens

PARTS USED   The stems, leaves, and seeds.

SIGNATURE   1. The thick, juicy stems.

2. The aromatic seeds. A transverse cutting at the base of this food displays a diaphragm-like characteristic.

SPECIFIC USE   1. The yield of a large amount of liquid from the stems caused physicians and herbalists of former years to classify the food as a diuretic.

2. This signature clearly states that the seeds—and the leaves and stems—are especially indicated in stomach disorders of all kinds. They are especially considered to be a warm aromatic and stimulating carminative, aiding in dispelling gas and wind in the stomach and calming the latter. Thus, we learn that the roots and stems were brewed in ancient times as a remedy for upset stomach, and now as a nerve tonic and sedative.

CENTAURY
Centaurium umbellatum, Erythroea centaurium

SYNONYMS   Bitter Herb, Red Centaury

PART USED   The dried flowering herb.

SIGNATURE   The deep rose-colored flowers.

SPECIFIC USE Used in blood disorders, it acts upon the liver and kidneys, as well as purifying the bloodstream.

AMERICAN CENTAURY
Sabbatia angularis

SYNONYMS Rose Pink, Bitter Clover, Bitterbloom

PART USED The whole herb.

SIGNATURE The flowers. They are of a rich rose or carnation color.

SPECIFIC USE Internally, it is for blood disorders. Externally, a strong decoction of the whole herb has been used to cleanse acne, pimples, and other skin disorders arising from impure blood.

CHAMOMILE
Matricaria chamomila, Anthemis nobilis

PARTS USED The flowers. Upper half of the plant.

SIGNATURE 1. The head-shaped flowers.
2. The herb, as described by the herbalist William Turner, "hath flowers wonderfully shynynge yellow and resemblynge the appell of an eye."

SPECIFIC USE 1. Its anticolic and carminative properties are well known, and indicate its employment in cases of cramps, flatulence, and other gastrointestinal disorders. But the signature indicates its use as a calmative and sedative in nervous disorders and headaches.
2. In combination with fennel and eyebright, chamomile has often been used as a lotion for sore, weak, or inflamed eyes. For this purpose, ⅛ teaspoonful of each herb is steeped in a cup of hot water, which, when cold, is strained carefully through

absorbent cotton. Chamomile has been used for this purpose since the early 1600s.

WILD CHERRY
Prunus serotina

SYNONYM   Wild Black Cherry, Choke Cherry

PART USED   The bark of the trunk.

SIGNATURE   1. The bark of young trees is marked with many white horizontally elongated lenticels.
2. The gummy exudation.

SPECIFIC USE   1. The lenticels indicate the astringent and healing properties of the bark, a decoction of which may be applied directly to external sores and cuts. A solution of the gum acts in a similar manner.
2. The shrub's exudations represent the exudation of the body and may be used for internal and external purposes. Internally, the gum, when dissolved in a suitable base, is used as a pectoral sedative in cough preparations, as is the officially recognized part indicated above. Its astringent action makes it valuable in catarrhal affections, whooping cough, and other bronchial disorders caused by the hardened accumulations of mucus.

CHESTNUT
Castanea dentata

PART USED   The leaves.

SIGNATURE   The leaf margins are sharp-pointed, thus indicating a pain- or paroxysm-relieving effect.

SPECIFIC USE   It is much recommended in cough remedies for whooping cough and similar irritations of the respiratory organs.

CHIVE
Allium schoenoprasum

PART USED   The edible portions.

SIGNATURE   The hollow stems.

SPECIFIC USE   Chives (as well as garlic and onion, and other members of its family) are indicated as a preventative agent against the harmful effects of toxic matter lodging along the bronchial and intestinal canals.

Chives and the related plants abound in blood-fortifying sulfur and iron. It is the sulfur component which is somewhat similar to garlic's active bactericidal crotonaldehyde, a worthy fortifier of the nasal and respiratory areas against infection. (Perhaps that is why garlic-eating Italians rarely are asthma victims.) Moreover, the members of the chive family stimulate the saliva and digestive juices while at the same time performing the duties of intestinal antiseptic. A syrup of chives (or of onion or garlic) serves well as a cold-cough remedy especially useful in croup or spasms of asthma.

CINQUEFOIL
Potentilla canadensis, P. reptans

SYNONYMS   Five-Leaf Grass, Five-Finger Grass (The seven-leaf form is Septfoil.)

PART USED   The entire herb.

SIGNATURE   The creeping, thread-like stems represent a needle-and-thread healing effect. (See also Septfoil, Gold Thread.)

A decoction of the herb has been found to be most effective as an astringent for internal and external purposes. A strong decoction is a good gargle for bleeding of gums and sore throats. The same solution may be used as a quickly acting remedy for diarrhea and bowel complaints. Externally, the cold decoction is also used to heal skin sores and ulcers, and to stay the bleeding of wounds.

CITRONELLA
Cymbopogon nardus, C. winterianus, Andropogon nardus

SYNONYM   Indian Nard

SIGNATURE   The habitat—the mosquito-infested wet areas where the herb either grows or is cultivated. (The herb is grown commercially in the wet lowlands of Ceylon, Java, and Malaya.)

SPECIFIC USE   The use of oil of citronella as a mosquito repellant is too well known to warrant further comment. This is an especially outstanding example of a remedy actually co-existing with the very cause that has created the diseased condition. (See also Eucalyptus.)

CLEAVERS
Galium aparine

SYNONYMS   Bedstraw, Clivers, Goosegrass

PART USED   The entire herb.

SIGNATURE   1. The herb grows in moist waste places and thickets and along the banks of streams.
2. Thin procumbent stems represent the needle-thread idea.

SPECIFIC USE   1. It is much valued as a strong diuretic and refrigerant in dropsy and in disorders of the kidney organs, upon which the herb also acts as an antilithic, to dissolve out gravel and stone.
2. The very slender stems display the herb's healing qualities. It is useful for sores, ulcers, and burns.

RED CLOVER
Trifolium pratense

PART USED   The flowering tops.

SIGNATURE   The rose-red colored blossoms.

SPECIFIC USE   The herb has enjoyed a long and well deserved reputation as a blood purifier. It is much used as an alterative and deobstruent in blood disorders, boils, pimples, and other skin eruptions.

CLUB MOSS
Lycopodium clavatum

SYNONYM   Vegetable Sulfur

PARTS USED   The entire plant, the spores.

SIGNATURE   1. The spore-bearing capsules located on the inner side of the bracts covering the fruit spike are kidney-shaped.
2. The trailing, branching stems that measure several feet long.

SPECIFIC USE   The herb was used as a diuretic in various kidney complaints and in calculous and dropsical disorders. Until recently, the moss and spores were employed as a nervine and antispasmodic in nervous disorders, epilepsy, etc.

COLTSFOOT
Tussilago farfara

SYNONYMS   Coughwort, Cough Herb

PART USED   The leaves.

SIGNATURE   The chief identifying physical characteristic of coltsfoot is seen when a handful of cut or ground leaves is pressed together: it stays in that pressed state. This observa-

tion may have led the Indian medicine men and the early herbalists to believe that the herb's active substance would attach
itself to the body's toxins. (This is true also of sage, hoarhound, and everlasting.)

SPECIFIC USE The herb is a well-known demulcent and expectorant and abounds in a mucilaginous extract that causes it to
be often included in cough syrups. (*Tussilago* signifies "cough
dispeller.") Combined with aromatics and other demulcents,
it has often been recommended for use in chronic bronchitis,
colds, and asthmatic complaints.

GARDEN COLUMBINE
Aquilegia vulgaris

WILD COLUMBINE
Aquilegia canadensis

SYNONYM Culverwort

PARTS USED Root, leaves, seeds.

SIGNATURE 1. It prefers chalky soil and rocks, and so has
become popular in rock gardens.

2. Its generic title is from *aquilegus*, denoting its water-
drawing and water-holding power.

3. Its glutinous seeds and flowers.

SPECIFIC USE The first two signatures would represent the
herb as a diuretic, capable of dissolving gravel and stone from
the kidneys and bladder. The sticky flowers are an indication
of its healing or astringent value, for irritations of the throat
and mouth, and for skin sores.

COMFREY
Symphytum officinale

PARTS USED   The leaves and roots.

SIGNATURE   1. The leaves are glutinous and rich in mucilage; when chewed gently, they will display that property.
2. The stalks are hollow.
3. All parts of the plant are covered with rough hairs.

SPECIFIC USE   1. Its action is similar to that of the mallows. It is an excellent emollient, demulcent, and expectorant in all cough remedies.
2. It is often used to remove catarrh from the tubes of the bronchial and alimentary systems.
3. The roughness of the hairs represents irritated conditions of the body, for which comfrey came to be used not only as a vulnerary and pain-relieving wash for inflamed or sensitive conditions, but as an internal remedy as well. The leaves were employed as mentioned above and are still applied as a hot fomentation to bruises and swellings and as a poultice to suppurating boils and raw, painful ulcers. Today's medical literature proclaims the merits of a substance known as allantoin, of which an appreciable quantity is found in the root of comfrey, and which for almost sixty years has been highly valued for its remedial service in ulcerations both external and internal.

PURPLE CONEFLOWER
Brauneria pallida, B. angustifolia

SYNONYMS   Rudbeckia, Black Sampson

PART USED   The root system.

SIGNATURE   The large, rose-purple, conical head of florets represents a boil.

SPECIFIC USE   It was much used as a remedy for boils, septicemia, and other blood disorders. The herb has been combined with burdock and red clover as a specific remedy to aid in the removal of blood impurities.

COWBERRY
Vaccinium vitis-idaea

SYNONYMS   Mountain or Rock Cranberry, Red Bilberry, Whortleberry

PART USED   The leaves.

SIGNATURE   The habitat, which is dry, rocky soil.

SPECIFIC USE   The small, dry leaves have diuretic and antilithic properties valuable in gravel and kidney complaints.

CRANBERRY
Vaccinium macrocarpon

SYNONYMS   Large, American, or Bog Cranberry

PARTS USED   The fruits and leaves.

SIGNATURE   1. The plants grow in rich bogs and marshes.
  2. The red fruits.

SPECIFIC USE   1. The leaves possess antilithic and diuretic properties and are useful in most kidney disorders. They may be used as a substitute for bearberry leaves.
  2. The fruits are said to be good for the removing of blood toxins and very effective in liver troubles.

CUCUMBER
Cucumis sativus

SIGNATURE   1. Note that this food contains 95–96% water and yields numerous seeds.

2. The green skin of the usual varieties shows small, scattered spines or soft, rounded mounds.

SPECIFIC USE   1. The cucumber is probably the best natural diuretic known. Cucumber juice added to carrot juice is of benefit in rheumatic ailments resulting from an excessive retention of uric acid in the system. With its high potassium content, cucumber is very valuable in correcting conditions of high and low blood pressure.

2. In former days, the cucumber served as the basis of many popular complexion lotions and emollient ointments and jellies. These preparations were much used, even in the early part of this century, to promote the healing of irritated skin. Cucumber jelly will also prove to be an excellent application for chapped hands, irritations, and roughness of the skin.

DANDELION
Taraxacium officinale

PARTS USED   The leaves and roots.

SIGNATURE   The yellow flowers.

SPECIFIC USE   The medicinal virtues of this most worthy herb have been long established. It is much used in catarrhal jaundice and in gallbladder and liver complaints.

DEWBERRY
Rubus procumbens, R. villosus

SYNONYM   Trailing Blackberry

PARTS USED   The leaves and fruits.

SIGNATURE   1. The stout recurved prickles borne on the stems.
2. The characteristic astringency of the roots.

SPECIFIC USE   Its uses are those of the blackberry.

DIGITALIS
Digitalis purpurea

SYNONYMS   Foxglove, Fingers

SIGNATURE   Its original habitat is said to be rock crevices, where it was first found growing. It is now well acclimated to all kinds of soil and is often cultivated in gardens.

SPECIFIC USE   It must be noted that this herb was at first used, not as a heart stimulant, but as a diuretic to eliminate stone and gravel deposits, and in conditions of dropsy, fevers, and inflammations. It worked so well that its beneficial effects upon the diseased heart apparatus also became apparent, since kidney and heart disorders are closely allied.

YELLOW DOCK
Rumex crispus

SYNONYMS   Curled, Sour, or Narrow Dock (Water Dock, *Rumex aquatica,* Butter Dock, *Rumex obtusifolius*)

PARTS USED   The leaves and roots.

SIGNATURE   The golden yellow of the roots.

SPECIFIC USE   Yellow dock is a strong alterative, deobstruent, and detergent, and today, as in past centuries, has served to rectify cases of jaundice, congested liver, and chronic gallbladder complaints. Up to the 1930s the herb was still prescribed by medical physicians in blood diseases, from spring eruptions to scurvy, and resultant skin disorders. Herbalists throughout the years have found it a good substitute for sarsaparilla in scrofula and glandular swellings.

DOG-GRASS
Agropyron repens

SYNONYMS   Couch, Witch, or Quack Grass

PART USED   The root system.

SIGNATURE   The long, smooth roots have been found to penetrate the fleshy roots of other much larger and far sturdier plants.

SPECIFIC USE   A decoction of the roots is considered a most worthy penetrant of clogged urinary apparatus, to help eliminate stone and gravel from the kidneys and the bladder. It is a thorough demulcent-diuretic and is especially useful in the treatment of cystitis and other catarrhal diseases of the genito-urinary tract.

DOGWOOD
Cornus florida

SYNONYMS   Flowering Dogwood, Cornel, Green Osier

PART USED   The bark of the root.

SIGNATURE   The external side of the bark is scaly or finely roughened.

SPECIFIC USE   The bark has antiseptic and astringent properties and has been employed, with other herbs, as a healing poultice for ulcers and erysipelas. An ointment may be prepared by boiling the herb in lard.

ELDER
Sambucus nigra, S. canadensis

SYNONYM   Sweet Elder (Dwarf Elder, *S. ebulus*)

PARTS USED   The leaves, flowers, and fruits.

SIGNATURE 1. The fresh stems are made fully hollow by pushing out the soft, porous pith (thus another synonym, Bore-tree).

2. It grows along borders of streams and in low, moist ground.

3. The yellowish-gray bark is marked by lenticels (fissures in the stem's epidermis).

SPECIFIC USE 1. The hollowing of the herb's stem represents the herb's medicinal action. Its stimulating-diaphoretic property effectively helps to push out the mucous deposits from the bronchial tubes.

2. Elder flowers are also of good service as a diuretic for minor urinary troubles and more popularly as a febrifuge in feverish colds.

3. The lenticels indicate the herb's healing property. The freshly dried leaves and flowers have been much used in creams, ointments, and lotions to allay itching and inflammation of pimples, acne, and other skin eruptions. A strong infusion of the flowers mixed with an equal amount of cider vinegar is similarly cooling and healing.

ELECAMPANE
Inula helenium

PART USED The root.

SIGNATURE The large yellow flowers.

SPECIFIC USE Its alterative and gently stimulating properties are indicated in hepatic torpor.

ELM
Ulmus fulvus

SYNONYM Slippery Elm

PART USED The dried inner bark.

SIGNATURE By chewing a piece of the bark, one will observe the property for which elm bark is so well known. The bark will yield a bland mucilaginous substance that designates the herb's medicinal virtues as emollient and demulcent.

SPECIFIC USE Well-known for the latter properties, it is much used in all catarrhal disturbances and irritations of the bronchial and alimentary systems. It is especially indicated in cough remedies as a mild expectorant to facilitate the removal of phlegm.

WATER ERYNGO
Eryngium maritimum

SYNONYMS Button Snake Root, Sea Holly, Rattlesnake Root

PARTS USED The roots and leaves.

SIGNATURE The herb dwells in mucky swamps and wet lowlands.

SPECIFIC USE It is an excellent eliminator of phlegm and other deposits from the body system. It first acts as a carminative in flatulence, to expel gas from the intestinal tract. The herb helps to stimulate a sluggish liver and the kidney tract in cases of dropsy and calculus. The leaves serve as a dependable diaphoretic and expectorant in bronchial disorders to facilitate the removal of phlegm.

EUCALYPTUS
Eucalyptus globulus

SYNONYMS Blue Gum Tree, Fever Tree

PARTS USED The leaves, the oil, and the gum.

SIGNATURE A large tree, it grows best in valleys having a rich, moist soil. In many semi-tropical countries it has been intro-

duced because of its reputation as a means of drying up miasmatic bogs. Because of its strongly antiseptic qualities, it is
today cultivated in malaria-infested areas and in unhealthy
swampy regions.

SPECIFIC USE   The fresh leaves are employed for the carminative and expectorant qualities, and the gum for its astringent
action in pharyngitis and laryngitis. However, it is the aromatic,
volatile oil that is today more commonly employed. Its anti-
septic-stimulant properties are well noted in the treatment of
typhoid and malaria. The druggist has included it in remedies
intended to clear up the usual catarrhal discharges of the nose,
throat, and bronchial passages.

EYEBRIGHT
Euphrasia officinalis

PART USED   The herb.

SIGNATURE   1. The white flowers streaked with purple ex-
hibit a lower lip whose central lobe is yellow and gets darker
towards the center, thus suggesting the human eye.
   2. The numerous seeds that fill the small oblong fruit pod.

SPECIFIC USE   1. The herb has long been known for its use in
the usual diseases of the eyes. Tragus, Fuchsius, Dodoens, and
other great herbalists of the sixteenth century regarded eyebright as a specific in all general diseases of the eyes. In England
it is much used by lay folk and herbalists in eye remedies. In
Scotland, an infusion in warm diluted milk is dropped into weak
and inflamed eyes, and in Iceland, the folk use the expressed
juice of the herb. The French call it *casse-lunette* and the Ger-
mans *Augentröst*, "consolation of the eyes." The herb is called
euphrasy in the writings of Milton, Thomson, Spenser, and
other poets.
   Symptomatically, a jaundiced eye has represented liver dis-

orders; thus that organ was gently activated with decoctions of the herb.

2. The seeds indicate the plant's use in all mucous diseases where there is a tendency towards gravel or stone formation in the kidney apparatus or gallbladder.

FENNEL
Foeniculum vulgare

PARTS USED   All parts.

SIGNATURE   1. The seeds.
2. The yellow flowers.

SPECIFIC USE   1. The sweet anise-like odor and taste of the seeds are much used to season oily fish to prevent indigestion, since, as Culpepper correctly stated, "it consumes the phlegmatic humours which fish most plentifully afford and annoy the body with, though few that use it know wherefore they do it." Therapeutically, the seeds are considered a most gratifying aromatic, a gentle stimulant, and an effective carminative, and have been employed for colic pains and nervous stomach complaints. Only a very few years ago, a proprietary Elixir of Catnip and Fennel was much used for infantile colic.

2. The flat terminal umbels bear the golden-yellow flowers, a color which told the observant herbalist-naturalist that fennel was to be used in cases of jaundice and associated liver disorders.

FENUGREEK
Trigonella foenum-graecum

SYNONYM   Greek Hay-Seed

PART USED   The seeds.

SIGNATURE   The seeds yield much mucilage.

SPECIFIC USE   A thick paste prepared by soaking them in water yields emollient effects—internally, to soothe inflamed conditions of the stomach and intestines, and externally, to poultice wounds and inflamed areas.

MALE FERN
Dryopteris filix-mas

SYNONYMS   Aspidium, European Fern (American Fern, *Dryopteris marginalis*)

PARTS USED   The root system. The oleoresin.

SIGNATURE   In spring one observes the young leaves yet uncurled, growing as circular masses of undeveloped fronds, somewhat shaped like a curled-up snake or worm.

SPECIFIC USE   The extract of male fern, oleoresin, has been employed as a vermifuge (worm expellant) since the days of Theophrastus and Dioscorides.

FEMALE FERN
Asplenium filix-foemina

PART USED   The root system.

SIGNATURE   See Male Fern.

SPECIFIC USE   Especially because of this signature did the Cherokee Indians use this and several other varieties of fern as a specific remedy for worms: cinnamon fern, bladder fern, maidenhair fern, and Christmas fern.

FIG
Ficus carica

This succulent fruit has been greatly valued from the earliest times, as a food and as a medicine. Biblical references tell of its use as a boil remedy. The Greeks considered it an invaluable and basic part of the dietary for their Spartans and for the athletes, the latters' meals at times consisting only of that food. Pliny, Ovid, and Homer testify that the Romans encouraged the eating of figs, and other references by Dioscorides and Theophrastus would indicate a major role in Roman mythology.

PART USED   The fruit.

SIGNATURE   1. The ripened pear-shaped fruit resembles a maturing boil.

2. When the fruit, which is rich in sugar, is cut and soaked in warm water, a fairly thick syrup is produced which indicates its use in the removal of catarrh from the bronchial and alimentary tracts.

SPECIFIC USE   1. Cut into two and steeped for two to three minutes in hot water, the soft interior forms an excellent poultice for an abscess or inflammatory, maturing boils, or as an application to a gum boil. It is interesting to note that this food was used as a remedy for boils by Hezekiah over 2,400 years ago.

2. The juice obtained by soaking or stewing figs is said to be a remedy for a simple sore throat or cough, temporary constipation, and disturbances of the digestive tract. Its effective, demulcent action is most noticeable in treating catarrhal conditions of the nose, throat, and chest. Because of its mild laxative action, again helping to eliminate harmful catarrh, the fig was (and still is) included in laxative syrups, combined with senna and carminatives.

FIGWORT
Scrophularia nodosa and varieties

SYNONYMS   Knobby Figwort, Carpenter's Square, All Square Stalk

PARTS USED   The leaves and root.

SIGNATURE   1.   It is often found in moist places, such as damp woods.
2.   The dark blood-red flowers.
3.   The knotty tuberous roots.

SPECIFIC USE   1 & 2.   The usable parts have served as a diuretic in kidney disorders, and offer their remarkable depurative property in cases of skin and blood diseases and especially painful lymphatic swelling or scrofula.
3.   The herb is a well-established vulnerary. The leaves or a strong decoction of the roots are applied directly to inflamed swellings and bruises and all eruptive conditions of the skin.

BLUE FLAG
Iris versicolor, I. virginica

SYNONYMS   Flag Lily, Water Flag

PARTS USED   The rhizome and roots.

SIGNATURE   The plant is found growing in swamps, in moist areas, and on banks of brooks.

SPECIFIC USE   Its well-known laxative-diuretic action serves to cleanse the catarrh from the linings of the stomach, intestines, and kidneys. It is therefore also useful as a stimulant to a torpid liver.

SWEET FLAG
Acorus calamus

SYNONYMS   Myrtle Flag, Sweet Root, Sweet Cinnamon, Sweet Rush

PART USED   The roots.

SIGNATURE   1.   The herb grows in wet lowlands and swamps.

2. Internally the roots are pale orange to weak yellowish orange.

3. The root's surface has small, slightly raised root-scars which resemble the knuckles or joints.

SPECIFIC USE 1. Sweet flag has long been known as an active and thorough remedy for colic and dyspepsia, in which catarrh and gas must be removed. The herb's properties are aromatic bitter and carminative.

2. These medicinal virtues help the liver rid itself of the impurities that impair its proper functions. One important function is to store the unused carotene content which is converted into vitamin A; when this does not occur, the eyes suffer. It is interesting to note that the generic name, *Acorus*, is derived from the Greek *àcoron* or *coreon*, the pupil of the eye, diseases of which were treated by the ancients with this plant.

3. Sweet flag, more often mixed with other toxin-eliminating herbs than used alone, has been so indicated as a remedy in rheumatic complaints.

FLAXSEED
Linum usitatissimum

SYNONYM Linseed

SIGNATURE The seeds, soaked in water, yield an active constituent, a gummy extract.

SPECIFIC USE Because of the seeds' emollient and demulcent properties, they are used as a laxative and as a pectoral in colds and coughs, to remove harmful catarrh from the alimentary and bronchial canals.

FORGET-ME-NOT
Myosotis palustris

SYNONYMS Snake Grass, Scorpion Grass

PART USED The herb.

SIGNATURE   1. The synonyms result from a resemblance of the curled flower heads to the tail of a scorpion or small snake.

2. It abounds in wet lowlands, brooks, and marshes.

SPECIFIC USE   1. Herbalist Gerard wrote: "Dioscorides noted that the leaves applied . . . are a present remedy against the stinging of scorpions, and likewise boyled in wine and drunke, prevails against the said bitings as also of adders, snakes and such venomous beasts. Made in an unguent with oil, wax and a little gum, they are profitable against such hurts as require an healing medicine."

2. It has been much used in European countries as a mucus-remover from the respiratory organs, for which the herb has a strong affinity.

FRINGE TREE
Chionanthus virginicus

SYNONYMS   Flowering Ash, Old Man's Beard

PART USED   The root bark.

SIGNATURE   The internal surface of the bark is yellowish brown.

SPECIFIC USE   Its properties are aperient, alterative, and slightly diuretic. It has a most beneficial action upon the gall-bladder and liver and was formerly much employed in child-hood jaundice and to prevent the formation of gallstones.

FUMITORY
Fumaria officinalis

PART USED   The herb.

SIGNATURE   The small flowers are of a pale red or pinkish color, topped with purple, and yield a yellow dye. The small root is yellow.

SPECIFIC USE The *U.S. Dispensatory* declares the plant "gently tonic, alterative, and, in large doses, laxative and diuretic." Yet it has been employed for many centuries for its chief action upon the liver, gallbladder, and bloodstream.

GALANGA
Alpina officinarum

SYNONYMS   Chinese Root, Alpinia Root

PART USED   The roots.

SIGNATURE   1. The irregularly branched roots, marked with the five annual scars, present another instance, as with sweet flag root, of a knobbed form.
2. The external color of the root is cinnamon-brown, and the internal, yellow or orange brown.

SPECIFIC USE   1. The root is an ingredient of anti-rheumatic mixtures. It has been often used for foot pains.
2. Its stimulating and aromatic properties, plus the signature of color, have caused the herb to be much used in cases of liver and gallbladder disorders.

GARLIC
Allium sativum, A. canadense

PARTS USED   The leaves and bulbs ("cloves").

SIGNATURE   The long, grass-like, tubular leaves.

SPECIFIC USE   The food exhibits its therapeutic value especially along the bronchial, alimentary, and urinary systems, which, too, are declared to be "hollow." It is also called for in diseases of the nasal passages. Garlic is considered a most valuable medicinal, both as a preventative against possible infection and then as a curative when needed. It is an excellent intestinal antiseptic and an especially good but gentle stimulant to the digestive system.

GENTIAN
Gentiania lutea

PART USED   The roots.

SIGNATURE   The bright orange-yellow flowers and the orange roots.

SPECIFIC USE   It is an aid in jaundice and liver disorders, in which its stomachic and tonic properties help greatly to overcome indigestion and dyspepsia.

WILD GERANIUM
Geranium maculatum

SYNONYMS   Herb Robert, Cranesbill, Wild Alum Root, American Kino

PARTS USED   The roots. The leaves.

SIGNATURE   The colorful red hue displayed by the fading leaves.

SPECIFIC USE   It is a well-known styptic and astringent. A decoction is an effective remedy for both inward and outward purposes: for bleeding gums, sore throat, and internal ulcers, and as an application to infectious sores, bleeding wounds, and indolent ulcers.

WILD GINGER
Asarum canadense

SYNONYMS   Canada Snakeroot, Indian Ginger

PART USED   The roots.

SIGNATURE   1. The leaves, usually two in number, are kidney-shaped.

2. The plant's habitat is one of rich woodlands or in shade where the soil retains its even moistness.

SPECIFIC USE   1. The action is upon the kidney system, from which the herb helps to eliminate viscid matter.

2. The herb is a stimulant, aromatic, diaphoretic, and diuretic.

GINSENG
Panax quinquefolia

SYNONYMS   Man's Health, Five Fingers

PART USED   The roots.

SIGNATURE   The forked root often assumes the shape of the human form.

SPECIFIC USE   The name *panax* is taken from the Greek *panakas*, "a panacea," in reference to the many wondrous properties ascribed to the herb by the Chinese and Koreans. These people have employed the plant for ages and place a very high value on it as a near cure-all. It is a powerful restorative and is said to prolong life. The Chinese extol it for all disorders of the stomach, nerves, and lungs, and as a tonic to the five viscera. In this country it has been used as a mild stomach tonic and stimulant in digestive problems.

GLADIOLUS
Gladiolus communis

SYNONYM   Sword Flag

PART USED   The leaves.

SIGNATURE   The erect blades were supposed to represent the phallus as the symbol of the male organ of generation.

SPECIFIC USE   This feature helped to indicate the herb's therapeutic property. Not only were the sword-shaped leaves to serve
as an aphrodisiac; they provided an invigorating tonic and
gladiatorial strengthening effects. This herb's name evidently
was equated with the Latin *gladius*, "sword."

GOAT'S BEARD
Tragopogon pratensis

SYNONYM   Noon Flower

PART USED   The whole plant.

SIGNATURE   The golden-yellow florets.

SPECIFIC USE   The freshly expressed juice of the young plants
has been considered in gallbladder complaints as one of the best
dissolvents of gallstones.

GOLDENROD
Solidago virga-aurea

SYNONYMS   Woundwort, Aaron's Rod

PART USED   The leaves and flowers.

SIGNATURE   The habitat—dry, gravelly, or granitic soil.

SPECIFIC USE   Its use as a diuretic for gravel and urinary obstructions has long been acclaimed by herbalists. Various species
have been of medical interest because their pollen is a frequent
excitant, if a minor one, of hay fever. The plants are needlessly
avoided because many sufferers are "allergic" to the pollen, but
actually the goldenrod is one of the most useful medicines we
have in the treatment of hay fever.

GOLDENSEAL
Hydrastis canadensis

SYNONYMS   Yellow Root, Yellow Puccoon

PART USED   The roots.

SIGNATURE   1. The plant is found in shady woods and wet places.
2. The red fruits. The yellowish roots.

SPECIFIC USE   Our North American Indians considered this herb a most valuable stomachic and application for sore eyes. They used it for various purposes long before the discovery of America. The underground portion was employed as a dye and as an internal remedy and soon became quite invaluable to the early settlers.
1. The herb's alterative and cleansing action is indicated in catarrhal disturbances of the stomach and colon and takes place especially along the mucous membranes.
2. These two signatures indicate a combined action upon the bloodstream, the liver, and the gallbladder. Goldenseal is a safe and reliable tonic in dyspepsia, stomach catarrh, and liver disorders.

GOLD THREAD
Coptis greenlandica

SYNONYMS   Canker or Mouth Root, Yellow Root

PART USED   The whole plant.

SIGNATURE   1. The intense yellow color.
2. The long, thread-like roots designate healing.

SPECIFIC USE   1. It is often combined with other antidyspeptic herbs (rhubarb, sweet flag, gentian) for disorders of the liver and gallbladder. Its chief constituent, berberine, is present also in barberry and goldenseal, thus permitting substitution for either.

2. The thin spreading root yields a needle-thread effect, to heal (as if to sew together) mouth lesions or cankers. It has an excellent reputation as an astringent wash for mouth sores, gum boils, and external ulcers. A decoction provides a good gargle for sore throat.

GOOSEBERRY
Ribes oxyacanthoides

SYNONYMS   Groser, Feverberry

PARTS USED   The fruits and leaves.

SIGNATURE   1. The habitat—wet woods and swamps.

2. The scattered prickles. Consider the origin and significant meaning of *oxyacanthoides: oxys* meaning "sharp" and *akantha,* "thorn."

SPECIFIC USE   1. The herb is used for diseases of wetness, colds and fevers. The juice is also used in domestic medicine against catarrhs.

2. The prickles indicate the painful symptoms of the above situations.

GRAPE

SIGNATURE   1. The water content and seeds.

2. The long, winding vine.

SPECIFIC USE   1. These alkaline and mineral-rich fruits do help the body to rid itself of its accumulated toxins. They help greatly to decrease the acidity of the uric acid and to eliminate the acid from the system, thus immensely benefiting kidney function. Tartaric acid, and more often potassium acid tartrate, abounds in the darker variety of grapes, enhancing the diuretic action. A mono-diet of seeded grapes is intended as an aid in the more complete elimination of gravel and stone from the kidneys and bladder.

2. The freshly extracted juice has been employed as an effective blood fortifier.

GRINDELIA
Grindelia robusta, G. humilis, G. squarrosa

SYNONYMS   Gum Plant, Gum Weed, Tar Weed

PARTS USED   The leaves and flowering tops. Resinous exudation.

SIGNATURE   1. The large flower heads are resinous and covered with a glutinous varnish.
2. Grows in salt marshes.

SPECIFIC USE   1. Its extract is used locally for dermatitis and burns.
2. It is a useful stimulating expectorant and antispasmodic in bronchial disorders and catarrh, where there is a tendency to asthma. It is also a gentle kidney stimulant.

GROMWELL
Lithospermum officinalis

SYNONYM   Gromill

PART USED   The herb.

SIGNATURE   1. It grows in dry gravelly soil.
2. Its egg-shaped seeds are hard and stony.

SPECIFIC USE   To the observing naturalist the plant's habitat and physical description declared its use as a diuretic and dissolver of kidney stones. Such was the application in Elizabethan days when gromwell leaves were taken, steeped in barley water.

Europeans in those times also used the herb as a substitute for imported tea leaves. Perhaps drinking such herb teas led the Shoshone Indians in this country to discover the contraceptive action of a local variety, *Lithospermum ruderale*.

HACKBERRY
Celtis occidentalis

SYNONYM   Sugarberry

SIGNATURE   A combination of clues. As to its habitat, the herb is found in moist soil and gravelly areas. The deep purple fruits contain a large stone (seed), and a quartered pith.

SPECIFIC USE   These clues indicate hackberry fruits for urinary disorders, especially as an agent to cleanse the kidney tract and bladder of catarrhal deposits of stone and gravel which may lead to kidney stones.

HAWKWEED
Hieracium venosum

SYNONYM   Rattlesnake Weed (Devil's Paintbrush, *H. aurantium*)

PART USED   The herb.

SIGNATURE   1.   Because of the resemblance between the curious purple-veined markings of the leaves to the markings of the rattlesnake, the herb was believed to counteract the tear or the poison of rattlesnake bites.
   2.   The flowers, either yellow or orange-red in color.

SPECIFIC USE   1.   This resemblance would emphasize to the earlier herbalists the herb's astringent quality, for which purpose hawkweeds were thereafter used in eczema and skin diseases.

2. The plant's properties are stimulant and anti-bilious in liver and gallbladder disorders. (See Celandine.) It is a well-known medical fact that eye weakness may be originally associated with liver malfunction. Thus English herbalists recommend tisanes of hawkweed to strengthen the eyes, an ounce of the tepid liquid taken morning and night.

HAWTHORN
Crataegus oxyacantha
and other species

SYNONYMS   Bread and Cheese, Hagthorn

PART USED   The dried fruits.

SIGNATURE   1. This small tree may be found growing in gravelly roadsides. Its bright red fruits contain stony seeds.

2. The sharp thorns designate its employment in painful situations. The specific name, *oxyacantha,* is taken from the Greek *oxys,* "sharp," and *akantha,* "thorn."

SPECIFIC USE   It was formerly in great repute as a diuretic in dropsy, gravelly complaints, and in the usual kidney disorders. Its active constituents, crataegin and amygdalin (the latter is also present in wild cherry), were isolated and employed as a cardiac tonic and an aid in reducing high blood pressure, thus greatly helping to lessen the painful symptoms encountered in urinary and cardiac conditions.

HENNA
Lawsonia alba, L. inermis

PARTS USED   The leaves and flowers.

SIGNATURE   The small white and yellow flowers.

SPECIFIC USE   Aside from its popular use as a hair tint, it is much employed in the Near East and Europe for jaundice and liver trouble.

HOARHOUND
Marrubium vulgare

SYNONYMS Marvel, White Hoarhound

PART USED The herb, principally the leaves and flowering tops.

SIGNATURE The ground leaves, when pressed together, will stay in that clinging condition. The upper surface of the leaf is veiny and downy but it is the hoary undersurface that yields the characteristic.

SPECIFIC USE Hoarhound has long been noted for its catarrh-removing property in bronchial and stomach disorders. Prepared as a syrup, it is much used for coughs, sore throat, colds, chronic catarrh, and all bronchial affections.

HOLLY
Ilex aquifolium

SYNONYM European Holly (American Holly, *Ilex opaca*)

PARTS USED The leaves, fruits, and bark.

SIGNATURE 1. The leaves are edged with large, sharp prickles, thus signifying pain.
2. The viscid, mucilaginous substance obtained from the bark.

SPECIFIC USE The medicinal properties of holly, being diaphoretic and febrifuge, signify its employment in painful pleurisy and bronchial catarrh. It has also been heralded as a substitute for cinchona, the source of quinine in the treatment of intermittent fever.

HOLLYHOCK
Althea rosea

PARTS USED　The leaves and roots.

SIGNATURE　Its well-known mucilaginous property becomes evident when either the leaf or root is chewed. For this reason it is a permissible substitute for the "officially" recognized ground and marsh mallows.

SPECIFIC USE　Its medicinal properties are emollient and demulcent. The herb serves well in cough, laxative, and kidney remedies where there is need to remove harmful gravel and catarrh. Even today, the people of Asia, especially China, still prepare hollyhock leaves for their meals—uncooked in salads and cooked in soups. Combined with sassafras leaves, these leaves also enter into Creole gumbo soup.

SWAMP HONEYSUCKLE
Lonicera villosa

SYNONYM　Waterberry

PARTS USED　The early leaves and ripe fruits.

SIGNATURE　The plant grows in wet, rocky areas, in swamps and bogs. The blueberry-like fruits are quite juicy.

SPECIFIC USE　The usable parts were at one time employed as a kidney stimulant.

HORSEMINT
Monarda punctata

SYNONYM　American Horsemint (English Horsemint, *Mentha sylvestris*)

PART USED　The herb, especially the leaves and flowering tops.

SIGNATURE　1.　The habitat—dry, sandy places.
　　2.　The odor, strongly aromatic.

SPECIFIC USE   1. Its kidney-stimulating action makes it a diuretic in gravel and urinary disorders.

2. Horsemint has very definite carminative properties, making a most useful remedy for flatulence, colic, and minor stomach ailments.

It is an acceptable substitute for peppermint, spearmint, and other mints.

HORSETAIL
Equisetum hyemale

SYNONYMS   Shave Grass, Scouring Rush

PART USED   The overground plant.

SIGNATURE   The herb dwells in gravelly, sandy soil and alongside railroad tracks. It may also be found growing in wet places.

SPECIFIC USE   It is an active diuretic, antilithic, and astringent in most kidney and bladder disorders, and is of great value in eliminating gravel and stone from the urinary apparatus.

HORSEWEED
Erigeron canadense

SYNONYMS   Prideweed, Canada Fleabane, Fleawort, Scabious

PART USED   The whole herb.

SIGNATURE   The name *Erigeron* signifies "soon becoming old" and thus indicates the herb's therapeutic application. So named, the plant became involved as a near cure-all, and as a general all-purpose health tonic. It was especially called for in degenerative diseases such as diabetes and kidney disorders.

HOUND'S TONGUE
Cynoglossum officinale

SYNONYMS   Dog's Tongue, Gypsy Flower

PARTS USED   The leaves and roots.

SIGNATURE   The taste is most mucilaginous. (The fact that both sides of the leaves are clothed in characteristic short, soft hair and are noticeably soft to the touch also gave rise to the herb's use as an internal emollient agent.)

SPECIFIC USE   As a demulcent and mild sedative, it is of good service in bronchial catarrh, coughs, and pulmonary complaints.

HOUSELEEK
Sempervivum tectorum

PART USED   The leaves.

SIGNATURE   1. Besides growing on roofs and porches of houses, where, once fixed, it spreads by means of its offsets, it will be found growing on stone walls and other rock-work.

2. The fleshy, succulent leaves permit the plant to act as a reservoir of moisture and to retain vitality in the driest weather.

SPECIFIC USE   1. The medicinal properties of houseleek, being refrigerant and diuretic, cause it to be employed, though mostly in European countries, in the usual feverish conditions and urinary problems. The juice of the bruised leaves has been employed by English householders as an application to burns, scalds and inflammatory skin eruptions.

2. Culpepper was quick to praise the virtues of this herb. Said he: "Houseleek is good for all inward heats. A posset made of the juice is singularly good in all hot agues, for it cooleth and tempereth the blood and spirits. . . . It easeth also the headache, and the distempered heat of the brain in the frenzies, or through the want of sleep, being applied to the temples and forehead."

HYDRANGEA
Hydrangea arborescens

SYNONYM   Seven Barks

PART USED   The roots.

SIGNATURE   1. The shrub grows along the banks of streams, in marshes, and in wet places. The name *Hydrangea* means "water-vessels," from the Greek *hydor,* "water."

2. The stem bark has a tendency to peel, thus the synonym Seven Barks, each successive layer showing a different color.

SPECIFIC USE   1. It is a gentle diuretic and antilithic. The action is upon the kidneys and bladder, on whose mucous membranes it provides a tonic effect, dissolving and eliminating stone and gravelly deposits, thus reducing inflammation of the urinary tract and relieving the pain following the elimination of those deposits.

2. The layer-upon-layer characteristic may be associated with the medical term *accretion,* which might describe accumulations of particles such as kidney stones.

ICELAND MOSS
Cetraria islandica

SYNONYM   Consumption Moss

PART USED   The plant (a lichen).

SIGNATURE   When the plant is chewed for a while, its mucilaginous property becomes evident.

SPECIFIC USE   Primarily, the herb has been much used as a demulcent in chronic catarrhal conditions of the bronchial and digestive organs. It is also considered an excellent nutrient in general debility and, until recently, served as a nutritious food for Lapps and Icelanders, and for the Indians of northern Canada.

IRISH MOSS
Chondrus crispus, Gigartina mamillosa

SYNONYMS   Salt Rock Moss, Carrageen

PART USED   The dried, bleached plant.

SIGNATURE   1. A close examination of this phallophyte will disclose its resemblance to the human bronchial system.

2. Mixed with hot water, the dried plant yields a thick mucilaginous jelly.

SPECIFIC USE   A jelly prepared from the moss serves as an excellent emollient to allay coughs due to colds. Not only is it useful in bronchial disorders; it is also called for in kidney and bowel disorders.

IVY
Hedera helix

SYNONYM   English Ivy

PARTS USED   The leaves, flowers, and fruits.

SIGNATURE   This is the well-known evergreen creeper which climbs by aerial roots.

SPECIFIC USE   Because of its tenacity ivy has been used as a remedy for pressure in various parts of the body, including inter-cranial pressure. Like the American ivy, it was used for innumerable diseases, from head to toe, internally and externally. Older herbalists recommended the flowers boiled in wine for dysentery, in butter to prepare a sunburn remedy, and the brown resinous exudation as a toothache remedy. Its principal property was its powerful influence upon the brain and nervous system.

AMERICAN IVY
Parthenocissus quinquefolia,
Ampelopsis quinquefolia

This is the familiar shrubby, woody vine, climbing so extensively and, by means of its radiating tendrils, supporting itself firmly on trees, stone walls, and churches. We use it as a ground cover.

SYNONYMS   Virginia Creeper, False Grape, American Woodbine, Wild Woodvine

PART USED   The long, winding stems.

SIGNATURE   1. The vine here represents the bloodstream.
2. A moderate decoction of the stems and leaves demonstrates the mucilaginous property of the plant.

SPECIFIC USE   1. Its alterative and cleansing properties are indicated in scrofula and blood disorders.
2. The herb has been used as an expectorant in bronchitis and pulmonary complaints.

JACK-IN-THE-PULPIT
Arum triphyllum

SYNONYMS   Wild Turnips, Dragon Root, American Arum

PART USED   The bulbous root.

SIGNATURE   The habitat—wet or mucky soil.

SPECIFIC USE   The roots are much used as an expectorant and diaphoretic in asthma, chronic bronchitis, and catarrhal situations.

JEWEL WEED
Impatiens biflora

SYNONYMS   Balsam Weed, Touch-Me-Not, Wild Balsam, Wild Celandine

PART USED   The herb.

SIGNATURE   1. The orange-yellow flowers.

2. The habitat is one of rich, wet soil, and the herb is most succulent.

3. The swollen joints of the plant.

SPECIFIC USE   1. Small doses of the freshly dried herb may be used as a laxative stimulant to the liver, in cases of torpidity or jaundice.

2 & 3. It is here indicated in dropsical conditions and in disorders of the urinary organs. (See also Knot Grass.)

JOE-PYE WEED
Eupatorium purpureum

SYNONYMS   Purple Boneset, Gravelroot, Trumpet Weed, Swamp Root, Queen-of-the-Meadow Root

PART USED   The entire herb, principally the roots.

SIGNATURE   The plant grows in swamps, meadows, and rich lowlands.

SPECIFIC USE   Its efficacy as a diuretic in dropsy, strangury, and gravel is well known, thus its common synonym, Gravelroot. It has been used to a great extent in all chronic urinary disorders, gout, and cystitis. It may be used as a substitute for (white) boneset or when added aid is required to remove catarrhal deposits from the alimentary and kidney canals.

JUNIPER
Juniper communis and the variety *depressa*

SYNONYM   Horse Savin Berries

PART USED   The ripe fruits.

SIGNATURE   The habitat is one of dry or limestone hills. The immediate area consists of sand and stone.

SPECIFIC USE   Juniper fruits are recommended as a valuable stimulating diuretic in cystitis and as an aid in eliminating stone and catarrhal deposits from the urinary system.

KELP
Fucus vesiculosis

SYNONYMS   Bladder Wrack, Sea-Wrack, Black Tang

PART USED   The herb (frond or thallus).

SIGNATURE   The "swollen glands" situated along the "neck" of the frond indicated the herb's action upon the swelling goiter.

SPECIFIC USE   Concentrates or derivatives of kelp have long been employed in obesity, principally because of the iodine content. (The modern physician, having discarded to a great degree the staining "old-fashioned" solution of iodine, now prescribes the clear, colorless solution of potassium iodide.) Similarly, because of a resemblance between the swollen receptacles and scrofula, psoriasis, and other such "skin raisings," the herb was much sought after as an alterative and blood-purifying remedy.

KIDNEY WORT
Cotyledon umbilicus

SYNONYMS   Wall Pennywort, Wall Pennyroyal

PART USED   The leaves. These are circular, similar to nasturtium, and penny-shaped, thus its synonyms.

SIGNATURE   1. It is a most succulent plant.
2. It is found growing among moist rocks and in stone walls.

SPECIFIC USE   The leaves are cooling and diuretic and serve as a quick-acting remedy for diseased kidneys. Culpepper and his herb-using contemporaries employed the juice or distilled water for gravel and stone.

KNOT GRASS
Polygonum aviculare

SYNONYMS   Wild Buckwheat, Birdstongue, True Knotweed, Nine Joints

PART USED   The herb.

SIGNATURE   1.   This herb inhabits the banks of ponds, brooks, and other wet areas. It is also found in rich waste places.

2.   The generic name, *Polygonum,* is translated "many joints."

SPECIFIC USE   1.   A decoction of the whole herb is an effective diuretic and antilithic, and is most useful in urinary disorders to help expel the formations of stone and gravel.

2.   To the old-time herbalists the swollen joints of knot grass indicated swollen joints of the body and thus it was much used in arthritic situations. (See Jewel Weed.)

JAPANESE KNOTWEED
Polygonum cuspidatum

SYNONYM   American Bamboo Shoots

PART USED   The young shoots.

SIGNATURE   Their fast and amazingly prolific growth offers an abundant supply from spring to early summer.

SPECIFIC USE   The early growth (6–8 inches), as with other fast-growing herbs such as knot grass, dandelion, burdock, wild carrot, and peppergrass, should be employed as a worthy edible —in this case, an excellent substitute for asparagus.

LADY'S SLIPPER
Cyprepedium calceolus, C. pubesceous

SYNONYMS   Moccasin Flower, American Valerian, Nerve Root

PART USED   The roots.

SIGNATURE   The root and rhizome system of this indigenous perennial appears as a mass of thin, fibrous roots and was thought to represent a mass of spreading nerves.

SPECIFIC USE   The roots are considered a worthy nerve sedative and antispasmodic in mild cases of hysteria, irritability, nervous headache, and other nervous disorders.

LEEK
Allium porrum

PARTS USED   The leaves and bulb.

SIGNATURE   The long, narrow leaves of this hardy biennial are hollow.

SPECIFIC USE   See Garlic.

PRICKLY LETTUCE
Lactuca virosa, L. scariola

SYNONYMS   Wild Lettuce, Opium Lettuce, Lactucarium

PARTS USED   The leaves and gum.

SIGNATURE   1. The prickles on the lower part of the stem.
2. The milky exudation.

SPECIFIC USE   The first signature is an indication of pain when one is eliminating the hardened catarrhal secretions or exudation (the second signature) from the bronchial system. It was known in ancient times that lettuce eaten frequently induces drowsiness. The gum prepared from lettuce is an ingredient of the popular cough formula, Compound Syrup Cocillana, in which its sedative properties help to allay cough irritations.

LEWISIA
Lewisia rediviva

SYNONYM   Spathum

PARTS USED   The leaves and root.

SIGNATURE   The mucilage that abounds in the plant.

SPECIFIC USE   The North American Indian considered this a noteworthy foodstuff and also dried and stored a large quantity of it for winter use when edible vegetation was at a premium. And when a simple mucus-raising remedy was needed, the mucilaginous principles of lewisia performed quite well.

LICHENS
various species

This is not a plant but a fungus found on the bark of trees, on walls and rocks. Its thallus (plant body) is described as crustaceous, membranaceous, and spreading.

SIGNATURE   The fungus bears a close resemblance to the skin disorder called psoriasis, which is defined as "a chronic skin disease, characterized by red patches covered with white scales."

SPECIFIC USE   A century ago, it was employed in the treatment of psoriasis, eczema, and other such symptomatic skin disorders. It must be noted that lichesteric acid, an antibiotic yielded by several lichens, inhibits the activity of the infection-causing staphylococcus bacteria.

LICORICE
Glycyrrhiza glabra and varieties

SYNONYM   Sweet Wood

PART USED   The root system.

SIGNATURE   The long horizontal rhizome (root) is sweet and slightly mucilaginous.

SPECIFIC USE   The signature of the root has long reminded the herbalist to use the roots as a blood remedy, as in the case of sarsaparilla and American vine. Recently, plant researchers found a hormone in the root which was efficacious in conditions of asthma, psoriasis, and blood disorders.

The saccharine, mucilaginous substance denotes the demulcent-emollient properties of the root. For centuries, licorice has been considered an effective remedy for dry cough and all bronchial disorders, noted as early as the third century B.C. by Theophrastus. It is also useful in the usual bowel and kidney complaints.

LIFE EVERLASTING
Gnaphalium obtusifolium

SYNONYM   Everlasting; Sweet, White or Field Balsam; Rabbit Tobacco (Pearly Everlasting, Cotton Weed: *Anaphalis margaritacea*)

PART USED   The herb.

SIGNATURE   As in the case of coltsfoot and hoarhound, the ground flower heads of everlasting when pressed together will stay clinging together.

SPECIFIC USE   The herb has been much used in cough syrup and gargles, and in pulmonary and intestinal catarrh. The signature shows the herb's action on phlegm or mucus.

LILY OF THE VALLEY
Convallaria majalis

SYNONYM   Muguet

PARTS USED   The flowers, leaves, and principally the roots.

SIGNATURE   1. The small, bell-shaped, nodding flowers were at one time used for the treatment of epilepsy, since it was believed that "that disease is caused by the drooping of humors into the principal ventricles of the brain."

2. It may also be that its original habitat was one of wetness, as indicated by its name.

SPECIFIC USE   Its continued employment for epilepsy may have witnessed a beneficial effect upon the urinary organs and later upon the heart. And its diuretic action, a usage which dates back to Aesculapius, may in turn have brought acclaim to its now better known heart stimulant property.

LINDEN
Tilia europea, T. americana

SYNONYMS   Lime Tree, Grass Wood

PARTS USED   The flowers and leaves.

SIGNATURE   The leaves and shoots are fairly mucilaginous, a property due to the gum and sugar constituents.

SPECIFIC USE   An infusion of the herb is taken to loosen and eliminate the catarrh formations from the bronchia and stomach.

LION'S FOOT
Prenanthes alba

SYNONYMS   Nabalus, White Canker-Weed

PART USED   The entire plant.

SIGNATURE   1. The exuding bitter juice.

2. The green-purplish markings of the tall stems, which the Indian herbalists believed bore a close resemblance to those of a snake.

SPECIFIC USE   1. The Chippewa doctor considered this a "milk root" and used the root as a remedy for female complaints, possibly as a douche in leucorrhea, to help arrest the discomforting white discharge of the vagina. At the same time a tea of the leaves was taken as a diuretic to flush the poisons from the urinary organs.

1 & 2. To the Indian, the oozing bitter juice also corresponded to the pus of a sore, for which purpose he applied a poultice of the leaves to the bites of snakes and insects. In time, the herb became better known for its content of the astringent tannic acid and was used not only in dysentery but as an everyday vulnerary, to heal cancerous and canker sores—thus the synonym.

LIVERWORT
Anemone hepatica

SYNONYMS   Liver Leaf, Hepatica

PARTS USED   The leaves and flowers.

SIGNATURE   1. From their similarity to the shape of the liver, the leaves came into use as a remedy for liver complaints. The specific name is derived from the Greek *hepar,* "liver."

2. An infusion of the leaves is mucilaginous.

SPECIFIC USE   1. The herb is a gentle remedy in liver disorders.

2. An infusion of the leaves has been employed in coughs and bronchial disorders.

LOBELIA
Lobelia inflata

SYNONYMS   Asthma or Emetic Weed, Indian or Wild Tobacco (Red Lobelia or Cardinal Flower, *Lobelia cardinalis*)

PART USED   The herb, after the seed capsule has opened.

SIGNATURE   The seed capsule becomes swollen, signifying the time to be collected and used as indicated, in all swellings and inflammations.

SPECIFIC USE   Lobelia has been used externally as a local hot application for swellings, sprains, and bruises. Internally, it was at first employed for such inflammatory disorders as tonsillitis and diphtheria but in recent times it has come into prominence as a specific for asthmatic and bronchial disorders.

LUNGWORT
Pulmonaria officinalis

SYNONYMS   Lung Moss, Jerusalem Cowslip or Sage, Spotted Comfrey

PART USED   The leaves.

SIGNATURE   1. The speckled or spotted appearance of the leaves was diagnosed as "spotted or diseased lungs."
   2. The infused leaves yield a mucilaginous substance.

SPECIFIC USE   It has long been employed as a demulcent and expectorant in bronchial and catarrhal affections. (Bullock's Lungwort is a synonym for Mullein, described elsewhere.)

MADDER
Rubia tinctorum

PART USED   The root.

SIGNATURE   1. The small, terminal flowers are yellow, and the root contains red coloring matter.

2. The prickly stalks appear very weak, for they are usually found growing prostrate upon the ground.

SPECIFIC USE   1. It was formerly used effectively in gallbladder, jaundice, and liver disorders. Madder has fallen into disuse because its red color is imparted to the milk and urine. As a source of red-to-purple coloring matter, it has always been held in high repute.

2. Madder was once used in rickets, a disease affecting the spinal column and the long bones.

MAIDENHAIR FERN
Adiantum pedatum

SYNONYMS   Rock Fern, Maiden Fern (Black Spleenwort, *Asplenium adiantum nigrum*, White Maidenhair, Wall Rue, *Asplenium rutamuraria*)

PART USED   The herb.

SIGNATURE   1. Since the fern is rolled up in the young plant but later unrolls and straightens out as growth takes place, a preparation of the fern was thought to help to unbend and straighten the constricted muscles of the rheumatic patient.

2. The habitat—rich, moist, wooded areas.

3. The thin, shiny stalks resemble a vigorous crop of hair.

SPECIFIC USE   1. The herb was well known for its anti-fever properties to the North American Indians, who employed it for initial rheumatic pains.

2. A habitat of wetness indicated its properties as an effective refrigerant in febrile diseases and intermittent fevers, and as an expectorant in chronic catarrhal and bronchial disorders. The lay herbalists include it in remedies for hoarseness and asthmatic disorders.

3. About 200 years ago preparations of maidenhair fern were much in vogue for the hair and scalp, especially in Euro-

pean countries. In recent years, the ashes of the fern were mixed with olive oil and herb vinegar and applied as a local application for alopecia.

MALLOW
Malva rotundifolia

SYNONYMS   Low Mallow, Cheese Plant (High Mallow, *Malva sylvestris*)

PARTS USED   The whole herb and roots.

SIGNATURE   The taste of the leaf is decidedly mucilaginous.

SPECIFIC USE   The mallows have demulcent and emollient properties and are indicated in all inflammatory and catarrhal diseases of the alimentary and urinary organs. Because of its mucilage content, the herb should be included in all cough and laxative remedies. (See also Hollyhock, Marsh Mallow, and Okra.)

MARSH MALLOW
Althaea officinalis

SYNONYMS   Mortification Root, Sweet Weed

PART USED   The root. The entire herb.

SIGNATURE   1. The sweetish root, when chewed, displays its pronounced mucilaginous property.

   2. This mallow resides in wet meadows, salt marshes, and on the banks of ditches and rivers.

   3. The stems are thickly clothed by a hairy down.

SPECIFIC USE   This herb was evidently in use in the early Greek period. Mallow is derived from the Greek *malake*, "to soften, to heal." The generic name is from *altho*, "to cure."

   1. The whole plant, especially the root, abounds in the

much-desired mucilage, which accounts for the herb's therapeutics as an excellent demulcent-emollient.

2. The herb's gummy matter serves admirably to soothe
irritations and inflammation of the alimentary canal and urinary organs.

3. This signature informs us that the herb will stop the
hoarseness or tickling in the throat and soothe and subdue the
pain of pulmonary catarrhs and general bronchial disorders.

MARSH MARIGOLD
Caltha palustris

SYNONYM   Cowslip (not to be confused with English Cowslip,
Primula veris)

PART USED   The whole plant.

SIGNATURE   1. These natives are found generally in wet
meadows, mucky swamps, and marshes.
2. The succulent kidney-shaped leaves.

SPECIFIC USE   1. It has pectoral and expectorant properties
which are helpful in loosening mucus and hardened phlegm from
the throat and bronchial passages.
2. The leaves were formerly employed by lay folk and
homeopathic physicians as a remedy for painful urination.

MASTERWORT
Heracleum lanatum

SYNONYM   Cow Parsnip

PART USED   The whole herb, especially the seeds and root.

SIGNATURE   1. The hollow stems.
2. The aromatic seeds.
3. The habitat—wet lowlands or moist soil.

SPECIFIC USE   1 & 2. The volatile oil of the seeds and the
stems indicates the herb's application as an aromatic and gentle
gas-expelling carminative, and a helpful corrective in simple
alimentary problems, such as stomach upsets.

3. The herb is a diuretic, often included in remedies intended
to increase the flow of urine and expel toxins and gravel from
the kidney apparatus.

FIELD MILKWORT
Polygala sanguinea

FRINGED MILKWORT
Polygala paucifolia

PARTS USED   The herb. The juice.

SIGNATURE   1. The exuding milk.

2. The plants are generally found in sandy and moist woods
and meadows.

SPECIFIC USES   1. At one time, milkworts were eaten by nursing mothers and fed to cattle, to produce a greater yield of
milk. (*Polygala* is from the Greek, "much milk.") But its true
intent is antiseptic, to heal broken skin and infected sores. The
milky exudation was also thought to quicken the removal of
deposits from the bowels and kidneys.

2. Its habitat of sand and moisture was indicated in kidney
problems and affections of the pulmonary area.

MISTLETOE
Viscum album

SYNONYM   Bird-Lime

PARTS USED   The leaves, flowers, and young twigs. The viscous
substance in the bark.

SIGNATURE   1. The clinging vine.

2. The viscous substance (birdlime).
3. The glutinous flowers.

SPECIFIC USE   1. Mistletoe is well known for its parasitic nature, having no roots in the soil but growing on all deciduous trees, such as apple, linden, pear, and hawthorn. The long vine clinging to its host was therefore regarded as the signature of the nervous system and was considered useful in all kinds of disorders of the nerve system. The medical compendia up to the early 1900s declared its use as an antispasmodic and nerve tonic, and for convulsive nervous derangements, especially epilepsy. Its choline content now permits an extract to be employed for high blood pressure and arteriosclerotic complaints.

2. The viscid material which gives rise to the synonym has been employed by the pharmaceutical chemist as a vehicle for many dermatological remedies, under the commercial name Viscin. Far more important, however, is the therapeutic property attached to *viscum,* which, translated as "seminal," referred to the viscid sap, which was formerly hailed as a therapeutic panacea, a cure-all. In Ireland and England it was much used as a revitalizer of the sex organs and so symbolized sexual survival.

3. The gluey nature of the leaves indicated their employment in healing sores and skin ulcers.

MOTHERWORT
Leonorus cardiaca

SYNONYM   Lion's Tail

PART USED   Upper half of the herb.

SIGNATURE   The sharp "thorns."

SPECIFIC USE   The stem is acutely quadrangular and at the intervals where once thrived the purplish flowers, there now stand guard the rigid and bristly "thorns," actually the de-

serted, bell-shaped calyx. The stem represents the spinal column, and the calyx, because of its five sharp awl-like teeth, pain.
(Sharp thorns or prickles offer a similar clue to thistle, hawthorn, and nettle.) In earlier days women who were prone to
headaches and menstrual pain used a warm tea of the herb to
relieve such discomforts, and found, as did the men, that it
served well as a strengthener of the nerve system and general
body tonic. It was formerly recommended also as a remedy for
amenorrhea.

MULLEIN
Verbascum thapsus

SYNONYMS   Velvet Leaf, Flannel Leaf, Velvet Dock, Candle-
wick Plant, Bullock's Lungwort

PARTS USED   The leaves and flowers.

SIGNATURE   Both sides of the leaf feel like velvet or flannel,
hence the synonyms. The wooly hairs on the leaf, like hoarhound's, indicate a tickling sensation of the throat and therefore of the bronchia.

SPECIFIC USE   Mullein has decided demulcent, emollient, and
pain-relieving properties, which have caused it to be much employed in coughs, asthma, and catarrhal bronchitis. Although
mullein's medicinal properties have been well respected for
some two millennia, there recently came to light the fact that the
herb may serve as an antibiotic source, inhibiting the growth of
various bacteria. Herbalist Gerard offered the leading clue
when he reported Pliny's observation that figs would not "pu-
trefie at all that are wrapped in the leaves of Mullein." For the
past century mullein oil has been an effective folk remedy
against disease germs.

NETTLE
Urtica dioica

SYNONYMS   Great or Stinging Nettle (Dwarf Nettle, *Urtica urens*)

PART USED   The upper half, especially the leaves.

SIGNATURE   1. The male and female flowers are found in the same panicle of the *urens* species and sometimes, though not usually, on the same plant of the *dioica*.
    2. The stinging hairs that cover the entire herb.
    3. A tall, lean plant with small leaves.

SPECIFIC USE   1. This is an all-purpose herb intended for all —male and female, old and young—to use. It has served as a most suitable edible for humans, animals, and poultry and entered many medicinal remedies.
    2. The sharp thorny needles designated its use as a remedy for "pins and needles," pleuritic and other stitching pains, and especially for arthritis. (Nettle juice, by the way, is a fast-acting remedy for nettle rash.)
    The plentiful hairs may also have caused it to be used as a hair tonic. Ever since the Middle Ages when nettle gained prominence as a food and medicine, it has been known to stimulate hair growth, and thus it is included in hair remedies to this very day.
    3. Not too well known is nettle's presence in reducing remedies, and in European countries, England especially, in the treatment for diabetes, there to cause a lasting reduction of health-harming pounds.

NEW JERSEY TEA
Ceanothus americanus

SYNONYMS   Red-Root, Mountain Tea

PARTS USED   Root or bark of the root. The leaves.

SIGNATURE   The large red root imparts a cinnamon-red color. The taste is decidedly astringent.

SPECIFIC USE   The astringency of the red color indicated to the early herbalists that the herb was required to heal the bloodstream. The *United States Dispensatory* informs us that "a proprietary tincture of *Ceanothus* (Ceanothryn) has been used to a considerable extent for the purpose of increasing the coagulability of the blood; especially for the prevention of hemorrhage from surgical operations." Indeed, the herb has been much investigated for its vasodepressing and other activity relating to blood circulation. Its astringency indicates the presence of a healing constituent, as yet undefined.

NUTMEG
Myristica fragrans

PART USED   The ripe seed.

SIGNATURE   The large seeds faintly resemble the scalp or brain.

SPECIFIC USE   In Civil War days, many grandmothers zealously guarded their nutmegs, which, being imported from a foreign land, were an expensive commodity. The seed was used as a remedy for insomnia: half a nutmeg, crushed and steeped in hot water, was taken upon retiring. The stimulating aroma of this warm spice, so prepared, also became a remedy for headache, though the grandmothers failed to realize that the cause, which the tea helped to overcome, was perhaps a combination of indigestion and nervous stomach condition. In small doses nutmeg is an aromatic stomachic and promotes digestion, but in large doses it is powerfully narcotic.

OAK
Quercus varieties

SYNONYM   Tanner's Bark

PART USED   The bark.

SIGNATURE   Many outgrowths, such as knots and excrescences, appear on the tree bark, the leaves, and at times on the early shoots.

SPECIFIC USE   This signature indicates external healing. The chief constituent of these abnormal growths is quercitannic acid, which is powerfully astringent and antiseptic. In the early colonial days its healing effect was used for skin irritations, inflamed sores, and indolent ulcers. Its astringency was also helpful in chronic mucus discharge and, infused with aromatics, in diarrhea.

OAK GALL
Quercus infectoria

PART USED   The galls, obtained from young twigs.

SIGNATURE   The galls are, and do represent, excrescences.

SPECIFIC USE   The galls have enjoyed long eclectic use as a healing agent, especially for skin diseases. They contain 50–70% tannic acid and 2–4% gallic acid, which are well known for their highly astringent and styptic properties. This latter mouth-puckering quality was well observed by Theophrastus, who employed it as a remedy for diarrhea.

OKRA
Hibiscus esculentus

SYNONYMS   Gumbo, Bendee

PARTS USED   The young fruits, leaves, and roots.

SIGNATURE The capsular, edible fruits of this annual abound in a mucilage (gombine) which is much used in the South to thicken soup and stews. The leaves and roots also contain much of this mucilage.

SPECIFIC USE The usable parts are employed wherever an emollient or demulcent is indicated. Once cut to a small size, it may be used as a sugar substitute to thicken a cough syrup or as a means of utilizing okra's mucilaginous property to soften up and eliminate harmful mucus throughout the alimentary, respiratory, and urinary organs. The leaves are used to a great extent as a healing poultice, while the long roots are often used as a worthy substitute for the scarce marsh mallow's, to which they are said to be superior. All parts of the okra, like holly-hock and the mallows, have the especial quality of softening and healing a diseased sore or external ulcer.

ONION
Allium cepa

PARTS USED The leaves and bulbs.

SIGNATURE 1. The long tubular leaves, a specific character-istic of the entire family.
    2. The concentric layers that constitute the bulb.

SPECIFIC USE 1. As with other members of its family, the quill-like onion greens are clearly specified as dealing with the hollow passages of the alimentary, urinary, and bronchial sys-tem.
    2. Ever since the ancient Egyptians noted that the onion was composed of layer upon layer adhering to its core, this food has been considered a means of having contagion adhere to the bulb and not to the patient. An onion hanging in the sick room was thought not only to keep additional disease away but to absorb the poison of contagious diseases which today we call

"pathogenic bacteria." Today we have proprietary mouth washes and lozenges containing the synthetic equivalent of the active bacteria-killing ingredient of onion. An effective cough syrup may easily be prepared by mixing the squeezed-out still warm liquid of a cooked onion with honey or a syrup of raw sugar.

The concentric layers of the onion also represent a condition of kidney stone formation which is a known act of accretion. The food, especially its greens, has been used for centuries in most urinary complaints: as a stimulating diuretic to increase the secretions and in gravel and dropsical complaints.

ORCHID
Orchis species

SYNONYMS   Salep, Saloop

PART USED   The ovoid tubers (roots).

SIGNATURE   1. The jelly-forming substance.

2. The tubers were found to be shaped like a testicle (from the Greek *orchis*, "testicle") or divided into two or three finger-like lobes. In mythology, the beautiful Orchis represented a cavalier of limitless passion.

SPECIFIC USE   1. The mucilage found in the roots produces a large quantity of jelly, requiring only one part to fifty parts of hot water. The substance has been much used in diseases of the gastrointestinal canal. Taken whole, the tubers are considered as nutritious as our potato.

2. Since early medieval days, the orchid's therapeutic properties have remained the same: astringent, nervine, stimulating tonic, and aphrodisiac. The latter is significant since the tubers were thought to act as a hormone-like rejuvenator for sexual impotence in the aging.

PANSY
Viola tricolor

SYNONYMS   Heartsease, Cordial

PART USED   The whole herb.

SIGNATURE   1. The herb yields an appreciable amount of mucilage and contains violine, a constituent similar to the emetine in ipecac.
2. The heart-shaped leaves.

SPECIFIC USE   1. The pansy was formerly employed as a demulcent and mild expectorant for bronchial coughs and asthmatic complaints.
2. In earlier days the flowers were in much repute as a good cordial for diseases of the heart. Perhaps, too, the popular name of Heartsease arose from their being an ingredient of love potions.

PAPAYA
Carica papaya

SYNONYMS   Pawpaw, Melon Tree

PARTS USED   The juice and fruit of the tree. The leaves.

SIGNATURE   The pale orange-yellow surface of the ripe fruit. The yellow milky juice.

SPECIFIC USE   The leaves and the juice of the fruit are in great demand in areas where the tree grows, in Florida and in most tropical countries. There they are used by the natives specifically in liver and stomach complaints, to overcome dyspepsia, impaired digestion, and gastric catarrh.

The Indians may have been the first to employ the papaya leaves as a meat tenderizer. Today, the enzyme found in papaya leaves is used in commercial meat tenderizers.

PARSLEY
Petroselinum crispum

PART USED   The entire herb.

SIGNATURE   Its habitat is the rich moist soil of gardens, but, more specifically, in shaded areas of walls and rocky areas.

SPECIFIC USE   The leaves and seeds possess carminative and diuretic properties while the sweetish root is regarded as more effective in dropsies and in eliminating various inflammatory conditions and gravel obstructions of the kidney passages. Note that the derivation of the generic name *Petroselinum* is from the Greek *petros*, "stone," and *selinum*, a parsley-like green herb. The ripe seeds, alone or as an extract, have been used in amenorrhea and dysmenorrhea.

PARSNIP
Pastinaca sativa

PART USED   The root.

SIGNATURE   The yellow flowers.

SPECIFIC USE   Until recently, parsnip root was used as a remedy for jaundice and disorders of the liver, from which it helps to remove obstructions. It also helps to ease the pain of colic arising from stomach disorders. However, it is a far better diuretic and should, along with the leaves, be consumed as a cleanser of the kidneys and bladder.

PARTRIDGE BERRY
Mitchella repens

SYNONYMS   Squaw Vine, Twin Berry

PART USED   The entire plant, especially the leaves.

SIGNATURE   The opposite round-ovate leaves.

SPECIFIC USE   As if to emphasize that the kidneys are on opposite sides of the spinal cord, so the leaves of this trailing evergreen have been employed as an astringent diuretic in most urinary disorders. A decoction of the entire plant has been used by the North American Indians, with raspberry leaves, to bring about easy labor in confinement cases.

PEACH
Prunus persica

PART USED   The fruit.

SIGNATURE   The soft down of the fruit. The kernel.

SPECIFIC USE   The down represented the hairs of the head. The kernels were boiled in vinegar, yielding a thick liquid which was rubbed into the scalp to stimulate hair growth and to "cure" baldness. Because the fruit's skin appeared to resemble human skin, the powdered kernels were substituted for almond meal as a softening agent for irritated, chapped, or inflamed conditions of the skin.

PENNYROYAL
Hedeoma pulegioides

SYNONYMS   Squaw Mint, Tickweed

PART USED   The herb.

SIGNATURE   It is an aromatic plant and has characteristics similar to other members of the mint family (Labiatae).

SPECIFIC USE   Pennyroyal, a gentle aromatic stimulant and carminative, helps to relieve nervous upsets or spasmodic pains of the stomach and intestines.

PEONY
Paeonia officinalis

SYNONYM   Pentecost Root

PART USED   The root.

SIGNATURE   Often the plant's rampant growth may cause the heavy buds to be top-heavy and to bend forward pendulously on their tall stems, almost falling down to the ground. The unopened buds appear to be shaped like the human head. Thus we are reminded of its therapeutic value against the "falling" malady, epilepsy.

SPECIFIC USE   Early in the history of Greek medicine, peony was prescribed by Apuleius as a specific remedy for epilepsy, as well as for mental and nervous derangements. Down through the ages, especially from the sixteenth-century Paracelsus down to the practising herbalist-doctors of recent days, peony root has been of great service in all nervous disorders, headaches, and convulsions. Today modern medical textbooks and compendia vouch for its antispasmodic property.

Furthermore, its anodyne property came into use during the 1700s as a comfort for teething babies—a necklace made of peony wood, similar in effect to paregoric or benzocaine jelly. Goldsmith refers to these peony anodyne necklaces in his *Vicar of Wakefield*.

PEPPERGRASS
Lepidium virginicum

SYNONYMS   Land Cress, Bird's Pepper

PART USED   The herb, especially the fruits.

SIGNATURE   The habitat—sandy and gravelly waste places and woodsides.

SPECIFIC USE   When the summer-collected aromatic leaves and fruits are used as salad ingredients or to flavor soups or other warming foods, one quickly notices the mild tang due to the highly alkaline minerals. For this reason, the herb is employed with other diuretics and refrigerants to remove stone and gravel from the kidney apparatus.

PEPPERMINT
Mentha piperita

SYNONYMS   Lamb, Brandy, or American Mint

PARTS USED   The leaves and flowering tops.

SIGNATURE   Wet or muck soil.

SPECIFIC USE   This herb has the distinct property of eliminating hardening mucus from the alimentary and bronchial areas and of preventing further discomforts of those organs caused by the mucus. Our early colonists and American Indian men often used warm teas of the herb as an antispasmodic stomachic and carminative for indigestion, colic, and flatulence. Combined with other herbs such as sage and boneset, peppermint was considered a worthy diaphoretic in colds, and a honey-sweetened tea of these three served as a cough syrup.

LESSER PERIWINKLE
Vinca minor

GREATER PERIWINKLE
Vinca major

SYNONYMS   Myrtle, Joy of the Ground (Madagascar Periwinkle, *Vinca rosea*)

PART USED   The leaves.

SIGNATURE   1.   The long trailing stems keep rooting and extending themselves in all directions and soon run riot, taking

almost full possession of the soil and surrounding area. (Horti-
culturists and landscapers have praised periwinkle's application
as a ground cover where little else will grow.)

2. *Vinca* is derived from the Latin *vincio,* "to bind," in allusion to its astringent and binding nature.

SPECIFIC USE   1. The rapidity with which it arrested hemorrhages of all kinds led to its specific use in tumor-cancer therapy.
Cancer cells are also well known for the runaway rapidity with
which they spread. That a periwinkle extract was to be considered for this purpose came to light in 1960 when an extract
of the plant known as vincaleukoblastine (VLB) showed promising value as an anti-tumor and anti-leukemia source of medica-
tion.

2. Because of its healing astringency, its "binding nature,"
the herb has been applied in lotion or decoction to all kinds of
skin eruptions, sores, and irritations and to some forms of
eczema. European herbalists prepare a periwinkle remedy for
long-standing cankers, inflamed tonsils, and ulcers of the mouth
and throat.

PERSICARIA
Polygonum hydropiper, P. opelousana, P. pennsylvanica

SYNONYMS   Smartweed, Water Pepper

PARTS USED   The leaves and stems.

SIGNATURE   1. The glandular dots give a spotted appearance
to the leaves of several but not all species.

2. The swollen joints, typical of members of *Polygonum*
genus. (See Knot Grass and Jewel Weed.)

3. The wet or swampy areas.

SPECIFIC USE   1. The spots gave rise to its trial as a remedy
for skin conditions. The plant was first used to heal pimples and
acne-like affections. Until recently it was simmered in warm

vinegar and applied to a gangrenous condition, and an infusion was found beneficial as an application to chronic ulcers and erysipelatous inflammations. Today we know of its antiseptic, healing property due to its content of tannic and gallic acids, a result which the early herbalists possibly did notice. Today we are quite aware of the antibiotic activity of the above three species: extracts of *hydropiper* and *opelousana* were found effective *in vitro* against *Staphylococcus aureus* and *Escherichia coli*, and of *pennsylvanica*, against the spores of *Neurospora crassa*, a fungus.

2. This feature caused it to be used for arthritis or joint swellings and gout. In Mexico and neighboring countries sufferers from rheumatism not only drink tepid teas of smartweed but soak themselves in a warm bath of the herb.

3. From this signature there developed its long employment not only as an effective diuretic in rheumatic conditions and as aid in removing gravel and stone, but equally as a good remedy for colds and coughs and the beginning of dropsies.

PERSIMMON
Diospyros species

SYNONYM   Date-Plum

PARTS USED   The fruits and tree bark.

SIGNATURE   The sharp astringency of the unripe fruit is immediately noticed when one bites into it.

SPECIFIC USE   The instant puckering suggested a source of fresh tannic acid to the herbalist who, perhaps already aware of the acid's healing power, thereupon began using it in diarrhea, chronic dysentery, and hemorrhage. In the days of the early editions of the *United States Pharmacopoeia* it was listed as an "official" drug and was prescribed by the medical physicians.

SCARLET PIMPERNEL
Anagallis arvensis

SYNONYMS   Weather-Glass, Red Chickweed

PART USED   The herb.

SIGNATURE   1. The red color of the flowers.
    2. The opposite leaves.
    3. The long, thin flower stalks, as they bear the glabrous capsules of the ripening seeds, tend to curve backwards.

SPECIFIC USE   1. The first two signatures are closely related. The first points to the plant's purifying effect upon the blood-stream and to the liver. So efficacious were the many virtues of pimpernel that it was held in high repute as a near universal panacea. The generic name, *Anagallis,* from the Greek *anage-lao,* "to laugh," was given by Dioscorides since it helped greatly to overcome the depression that accompanies or follows obstructions and disorders of the liver. With disease of this organ are associated those of the eyes; the Greeks first used the herb also for the latter purpose.
    2. The position of the leaves denotes the kidneys—hence its origin as an effective diuretic which would help eliminate gravel and stone from that organ. Almost fourscore years ago there was discovered in pimpernel an active ferment which tended, like papaya, to rapidly digest raw meat and so prevent degeneration of the kidneys and liver.
    3. This bending backwards led early investigators to consider the use of this plant in epilepsy. Its centuries-old reputation has survived in European countries where recent doctors have prescribed it in diseases of the brain. The dried flowers or the powdered leaves have both been found useful in epilepsy. Present-day doctors have found a tincture of the herb to be helpful in melancholia and related forms of mental disorders.

WHITE PINE
Pinus strobus and other species

SYNONYMS   Pinus Alba, Soft or Weymouth Pine

PARTS USED   The balsam, leaves, and inner bark.

SIGNATURE   1. The viscid pitch (i.e. the sap or crude turpentine).
2. The bark contains and produces the desired oleoresin (pitch) in blister-like cavities on the exterior of the trunk and thick branches.

SPECIFIC USE   1. The oozing pitch represents the rising phlegm or mucus which the body wants to eliminate from the throat and bronchia. Compound Syrup of White Pine and Tar is a mild, stimulating cough syrup that has outlived dozens of other proprietary remedies and contains the coarsely-powdered pine bark and other common herbs. Today it is still considered a demulcent, anticatarrhal expectorant, especially in coughs and bronchial discomforts, as well as in tonsillitis and laryngitis.
2. The crude pitch that appears on the round designs of knots or tree openings as well as on the sticky cones has been credited with healing sores and diseased openings of the skin. The oleoresin which is obtained directly from coniferous trees, and pine tar, a product resulting from the distillation of the wood of various pines, yield their strongly antiseptic qualities in various skin diseases.

PINK ROOT
Spigelia marilandica

SYNONYMS   Worm Grass, Indian Pink (Annual Worm Grass, *Spigelia anthelmia*)

PARTS USED   The rhizome and roots.

SIGNATURE   The numerous long thick rootlets gave an appearance of small snakes or large worms.

SPECIFIC USE   Carl von Linnaeus, the famous Swedish botanist
of the 1700s and the "father of modern systematic botany,"
bestowed the above botanical names. The *anthelmia* species
must have attracted his attenion for its special therapeutic property. Both species have enjoyed a good reputation as an anthelmintic (expeller of intestinal worms) and as a vermifuge (an
expeller of round worms). The name Indian Pink helps to remind one that the species was used by the American Indians
long before the discovery of our country by the Europeans.

PITCHER PLANT
Sarracenia purpurea

SYNONYMS   Fly Trap, Huntsman's or Water Cup

PART USED   The whole plant, especially the leaves and root.

SIGNATURE   1. The plant grows in wet, rich woods, bogs, and
swampy areas.

2. The dilated tubular leaves which constitute the pitchers
are often partly full of water.

SPECIFIC USE   1. The wet, spongy soil in which the plant
grows points to the herb's value in removing needless refuse
from the human boggy swamp, the stomach. Upon that organ
and the liver does the herb exert its cleansing, stimulant-tonic
influence. Often referred to as *nepenthe,* from the Greek "not"
and "grief," the herb was employed in ancient Greece to dispel
the temporary sorrow and misfortune which accompany the
discomforts of liver torpidity.

2. Equally important is its more specific use as a mild diuretic in urinary dysfunction. Water and water containing here
may be equated with kidney problems and their correction. The
American Indian held this herb in high regard for two other
reasons. Its leaves became his drinking cup when he was out
hunting in the woods or swamp, and the herb itself his highly
extolled medicine for sharpening his memory. The leaves are

well known for their singular habit of keeping anything imprisoned that has fallen into them. Here is applied the principle of sympathy: the herb was used to keep imprisoned in the mind the acquired knowledge.

PLANE-TREE
Platanus occidentalis

SYNONYMS "Sycamore," Buttonwood, Cottonwood

PART USED The bark.

SIGNATURE It inhabits streams and wet woods.

SPECIFIC USE The Cherokees use the tree bark as a quickly acting diuretic to relieve the painful symptoms in the hips and lower part of the back.

PLANTAIN
Plantago major

SYNONYMS Englishman's or White Man's Foot, Cuckoo's Bread

PARTS USED The leaves, fruits, root.

SIGNATURE 1. The mature erect flowering spikes were supposed to represent snakes.

2. When it is found growing in good soil, one notes that a span of two to four inches of bare earth encircles the herb. The plant has drawn from the soil and unto itself a great deal of the nutrients which rightfully should have been shared with other plant life.

SPECIFIC USE Plantain's resemblance to the snake, fancied or not, caused it to first be used to heal bites of venomous reptiles, then those of insects and later of animals. In our Southern states, where plantain is called Snake-Weed, when humans or animals are stung by a rattlesnake, a mixture of the concentrated juice of the herb and salt is applied to the wound, with good results almost guaranteed.

2. Plantain is an excellent vulnerary and astringent for external applications, to draw forth and remove felons and splinters, and to poultice boils and bruises. For recent insect bites, sores, and indolent ulcers, the leaves need only be crushed and dipped in hot water and applied to the affected area. The ubiquitous herb also offers its services as an antiseptic-magnet stimulant to the kidneys, from which the attracted toxins are removed.

RATTLESNAKE PLANTAIN
Goodyeara pubescens

SYNONYMS   Rattlesnake Leaf, Scrofula Weed

SIGNATURE AND SPECIFIC USE   Because its white-veined appearance was said to resemble a snake's belly, the leaves were considered an "infallible cure" for snake-bite and for external conditions such as scrofulous or eczematous eruptions.

POKE
Phytolacca decandra americana

SYNONYMS   Ink Berry, Garget, Pocan, Pigeon Berry

PARTS USED   The root, early shoots, and berries.

SIGNATURE   1. The hollow, succulent stems and berries.

2. The large fleshy root, which frequently exceeds a man's leg in diameter, somewhat resembles the human form. The main or upper thick portion equals the torso and is divided into similar but less thick branching roots which run deep into the ground.

3. The blood-red color that lodges in the stem and fruits.

SPECIFIC USE   1. Succulence of the hollow stems causes the herb to affect the organs of elimination, serving as a diuretic and laxative to cleanse the system of waste products.

2 & 3. These signatures obviously deal with the body as a whole and with the bloodstream in particular. The root's close resemblance to the human shape caused it to be used by Indian doctors as an alterative in organic disorders where other simples had failed or were not suitable. They taught the early white settlers the employment of the root as an emetic but more especially as a specific for rheumatism. Today, in herbal medicine, it takes first place with sarsaparilla among all alteratives. We are also aware of poke's chief constituent, which duplicates the action of cortisone, today's "wonder drug," in stimulating the entire glandular system. Thus, until recently, it was in great demand for the treatment of scrofulous and skin disorders, blood conditions and rheumatism, psoriasis and various skin problems. *A useful plant but to be used with caution.*

PRINCE'S PINE
Chimaphila umbellata

SYNONYMS   Pipsissewa, Bitter Wintergreen, Ground Holly

PART USED   The leaves.

SIGNATURE   1. Its habitat is one of loose, sandy soil, usually under pine trees.

2. It grows as a long, creeping evergreen vine.

3. The leaf margin is sharply toothed.

SPECIFIC USE   1. Sandy soil represents a gravel-stone condition of the body, especially of the kidneys, and for that purpose the herb has been considered quite applicable.

2. The nature of growth of this perennial evergreen, as with most vines or vine-like growths, emphasized its almost incredible power of penetration through and elimination of the

harmful obstacles from the kidneys and bloodstream. (See Dog-Grass.) Prince's pine has until recently served well as an astringent, diuretic, and mild disinfectant to the urinary tract and has also been recommended in cystitis and arthritic complaints. Indians and laity and physicians have used it in one form or another in all kidney, scrofulous, and rheumatic disorders. In the early 1800s it became a favorite remedy with the medical profession, anticipating the use of salicylic acid and the salicylates, which in structural form are constituents of this plant.

PRIVET
Ligustum vulgare

SYNONYM   Prim

PARTS USED   The leaves and stem bark.

SIGNATURE   The distinctly astringent taste of the usable parts.

SPECIFIC USE   A strong infusion heals spongy and bleeding gums, ulcerations of the mouth and stomach, and infected sores and scratches, and is also intended as a gargle for sore or irritated throat. It corrects also chronic bowel complaints such as diarrhea. Research scientists have discovered that three varieties of privet possess sufficient antibiotic principles to inhibit the activity of a pus-forming bacteria, *Staphylococcus aureus*.

PSYLLIUM
Plantage psyllium

SYNONYM   Fleawort

PART USED   The seeds.

SIGNATURE   The substantial amount of mucilage in the seeds.

SPECIFIC USE   Its demulcent and emollient properties declare its catarrh-removing effect in bronchial and stomach-intestinal irritations. Psyllium seeds are today used alone or included, as are their extractives, in laxative preparations.

GIANT PUFFBALL
Calvatia craniformia

PART USED   The inner spores.

SIGNATURE   An abnormal growth such as this fungus can be considered for healing purposes.

SPECIFIC USE   To quickly stop and heal nose bleeding, the Indians prescribed the powdered substance to be snuffed up the nostrils. Their midwives, after the cutting of a newborn's umbilical cord, placed a piece of puffball on the navel both as a prophylactic and as a therapeutic measure. Only a few years ago, cancer research at Michigan State University showed that an extract of giant puffball, calvacin, could arrest cancer in test animals.

PURSLANE
Portulacca oleracea

SYNONYMS   Portulacca, Pussley

PART USED   The overground portion.

SIGNATURE   1. This fleshy herb is well known for its exceedingly high water content.
2. The enormous number of tiny seeds.

SPECIFIC USE   Purslane's succulence and somewhat mucilaginous taste not only have increased its recent acceptance as a most wholesome food but have designated, since the days of the observant Pliny, its use as a cooling aid to and a cleansing stimulant of the kidneys and bladder in cases of strangury, scurvy, and urinary affections. The presence of the many seeds confirms this therapeutic value of purslane and helps to emphasize its especial aid in removing stone and gravel from the kidney apparatus.

QUASSIA
Picrasma amara, P. excelsa

SYNONYM   Bitter Wood

PART USED   The heartwood.

SIGNATURE   Its yellow color.

SPECIFIC USE   Quassia gained prominence about 200 years ago when a Surinam slave named Quassi disclosed that his secret and highly successful remedy for malignant fevers was based on the wood of the tree. Since then it has been equally commended in other situations. The intensely bitter wood is one of nature's best remedies against the formation of noxious substances in the alimentary canal resulting from the digestion process. Quassia's therapeutic action also prevents atonic dyspepsia and especially the overburdening of the liver. This herb has gained prominence among herbalists for its noticeable benefits to the eyes, probably by keeping the liver in good working order.

QUEEN'S DELIGHT
Stillingia sylvatica

SYNONYMS   Queen's Root, Yaw Root

PART USED   The root.

SIGNATURE   1. When the plant is broken, it emits a milky sap.
2. The yellow spikes of the terminal flowers.

SPECIFIC USE   1. In small doses, its excellent alterative action influences the secretory functions and therefore affects the glandular system. Up to forty years ago, the root and its preparations were extensively used for syphilitic and cutaneous disorders, for scrofula and leucorrhea. With aromatics, the root was found most beneficial in chronic catarrhal bronchial problems.

2. Queen's delight was found equally efficacious in liver disturbances.

QUINCE
Pyrus cydonia

PART USED   The seeds.

SIGNATURE   The distinctly mucilaginous characteristic of the seeds.

SPECIFIC USE   Plant mucilage removes mucus. In this case, the insipid seeds abound in a jellyish substance well known as an acceptable demulcent in coughs, hoarseness, and following feverish colds. For this purpose the freshly extracted mucilage is added (as is honey or brown sugar) to a suitable herb tea. This remedy is also especially indicated as a means of gently removing catarrhal deposits from and soothing an irritated or sick stomach.

ANNUAL RAGWEED
Ambrosia artemesiaefolia

GIANT RAGWEED
Ambrosia trifida

Here is indicated the doctrine of similars, that is, the principle that whatever causes a particular reaction or symptom will also alleviate or cure the distressing complaint. The modern physician, for instance, may assume that this plant's pollen is often the chief cause of hay fever and thereupon suggests the process of immunizing the sufferer with injections of minute doses of the disturbing pollen. It is interesting to note that long before the days of allergies and allergenic preparations, ragweed was employed as an astringent in cases of closed nasal passages and constant sneezing, so symptomatic of hay fever, and in similar chronic catarrhal affections.

RASPBERRY
Rubus idaeus

SYNONYM   Red Raspberry

PARTS USED   The leaves and fruits.

SIGNATURE   1. The red juicy fruits.
2. The numerous sharp thorns.
3. The taste of the root.

SPECIFIC USE   1. The fruits are an aggregate of about twenty small rounded and juicy drupelets which appear to be a tightly-packed accumulation of tiny accreted mounds. Better known for their delicious taste and nutritive values, they are accredited as a remedy for breaking up and helping to expel stone accretions from the kidneys and gallbladder. And their acidulous juice emphasizes their property of stimulating the urinary organs.

2. The stiff prickles indicate pain accompanying complaints of the internal organs. An interesting feature of this plant is the use of an infusion of raspberry leaves by Indian women during their pregnancy to facilitate delivery. Several years ago the name *fragarine* was given to the active principle of raspberry leaf extract which was used on a vast experimental basis in alleviating labor pains. The extract appeared to act mainly as a relaxant upon the uterine muscles.

3. The root's familiar astringency and well recorded healing properties have led to the discovery of the antibiotic value of several members of its family, which is due to a concentration of tannic and gallic acids. It has long been used as a gargle

for sore throat and cankers, as an application to bleeding wounds and cuts, and especially as a remedy for diarrhea and leucorrhea.

RATTLESNAKE ROOT
Polygala senega

SYNONYMS   Seneca Snakeroot, Mountain Flax

PART USED   The root system.

SIGNATURE   1. The milky exudation.

2. The root's concave side displays a projecting line that is usually twisted and somewhat spiral, like a snake.

SPECIFIC USE   1. The profuse secretion of milk is indicated in the name *polygala,* "much milk," and reminds us of the use of this perennial as an aid in the removal of mucus. Seneca has been employed as a diaphoretic to remove unwanted catarrhal deposits from the stomach and bronchial areas, and as an expectorant in croup, chronic bronchitis, and asthma.

2. The Seneca Indians used the root as a remedy for snakebite. The active ingredient of the root is a strong saponin capable of destroying pathogenic microorganisms. Several of the *polygala* family yield an aqueous extract which is effective *in vitro* against *Staphylococcus* and *Escherichia* bacteria.

RAUWOLFIA
Rauwolfia serpentaria

PART USED   The root.

SIGNATURE   A low climbing vine with a long snake-like root.

SPECIFIC USE   The dried root has been employed for more than three millennia in India for a long list of ailments, among which are bites of snakes and stings of insects. It is a good example of a climbing vine that represents to the signature-seeker a most specific remedy for the nervous system. Here, then, is another folk remedy that, given the proper laboratory research, has verified the initial therapeutics. The natives of India used it largely as a sedative for sleeplessness and as a near-narcotic to quiet the mentally disturbed.

Today's research has shown that the root does have strong sedative powers, does help greatly in insomnia without the dangerous side-effects of the barbiturates, and has been of great therapeutic aid in lowering blood pressure. Today's physician frequently prescribes either the whole powdered root or its more potent alkaloid, reserpine, for agitated patients and in the treatment of mild hypertension. Both forms have a tranquilizing effect upon the patient and at the same time cause a moderate fall in blood pressure.

COMMON REED
Phragmites communis

PARTS USED   The roots, early shoots, leaves, and seeds.

SIGNATURE   It is always found in areas of wetness, such as swamps, ditches, shallow water, and bogs.

SPECIFIC USE   The roots and seeds help greatly to increase urination and to diminish strangury and the presence of gravel from the kidneys.

ROSE
Red Rose, *Rosa gallica,* Brier Hip, Wild Brier, *Rosa canina,* Cabbage or Moss Rose, *Rosa centrifolia*

PARTS USED   The flowers, fruits, and leaves.

SIGNATURE   1. The natural habitat is sandy, gravelly soil.
  2. The many seeds within the fruits.
  3. The orange-scarlet color of the hips (fruits).

4. The odor and pollen often are rather irritating to the eyes.

5. The sharp prickles that cover the stem.

SPECIFIC USE   Signatures 1 and 2 indicate its well-known property of dissolving and gradually removing gravelly deposits and stone from the kidney and gallbladder areas.

3. The color represents conditions of the liver and bloodstream. A troubled liver may lead to serious derangements of the gallbladder and the bloodstream. These areas, and the kidneys, are indeed affected by the alkaline salts of the malic and citric acids which are also found in other members of the rose family, such as apple, pear, peach, cherries, strawberries. These ingredients constitute the "refrigerant" properties of these fruits. In Elizabethan days the distilled water of the leaves and flowers was highly praised for strengthening the heart and refreshing the spirits, and likewise for all things that required gentle cooling. Today the hips yield an equally important ingredient, vitamin P, which helps to prevent and to heal the rupture of minute blood vessels.

4. Rose water, once prepared from the flowers or attar (oil) of rose, is still used in several proprietary eye lotions, including those for relief of eye discomfort in hay fever.

5. The sharp thorns represent the pain that is associated with the above internal disorders.

ROSEMARY
Rosmarinus officinalis

SYNONYMS   Compass Plant, Incensier

PART USED   The herb.

SIGNATURE   *Rosmarinus,* the generic name, is from the Latin *ros,* "dew," "spray," and *mare* "sea," because of the plant's profuse weed-like growth in limestone along the Mediterranean coast. The plant grows best in stony or chalky places and especially in the light, dry soil of walls. In such a habitat, though a smaller height is produced, the oil is more fragrant and more concentrated.

SPECIFIC USE   The habitat of rosemary suggested to early herbalists its use "against obstructions in the viscera," especially of the kidneys. It then became a remedy for dropsy by stimulating the urinary organs. Not only was it successful as a freshly prepared wine or cordial to quiet an over-palpitating heart; it was considered exceedingly efficacious for headaches accompanying weak circulation. In time, rosemary tea became a good remedy in nervousness and nervous dyspepsia, sleeplessness, and head pains.

ROSIN-WEED
Silphium paciniatum

SYNONYMS   Compass Plant, Polar Plant

PART USED   The root.

SIGNATURE   From the plant there exudes a fragrant gum-like resin, which increases considerably in the torn herb.

SPECIFIC USE   The root has strong alterative and diaphoretic properties. It was considered an effective expectorant in dry coughs, asthmatic conditions, and pulmonary catarrhal problems. The herb was formerly used to relieve the heaves of horses.

SAFFLOWER
Carthamus tinctorius

SYNONYMS   American or Dyer's Saffron

PART USED   The orange-red flowers.

SIGNATURE   The yellow and red substances of the flowers.

SPECIFIC USE   The flowers are often substituted for the expensive saffron as a seasoning agent and have become a popular remedy for jaundice, torpidity of the liver, and gallbladder troubles, as well as a diaphoretic in eruptive maladies arising from an impure bloodstream, e.g. measles and chicken pox. Safflower has gained well-deserved prominence in recent years because of the fixed oil furnished by the seeds (25.8%) and their kernels (50%). Not only is this unsaturated oil now being used here for culinary purposes; it has been credited as a preventative medicine. By lowering the cholesterol level which has been too long under suspicion as one of the major contributing causes of arteriosclerosis and heart disease, unsaturated fats and oils like safflower's have been found to prevent possible damage to the liver, gallbladder, and the arterial system.

SAFFRON
Crocus sativus

SYNONYMS   True or Spanish Saffron

PART USED   The dark orange to red stigmas.

SIGNATURE   The color of the stigmas and their resultant yellow-red liquid.

SPECIFIC USE   Saffron's carminative-diaphoretic properties free the liver and blood systems from catarrhal formations and toxins that may accumulate along these areas. The herb is a gentle stimulant and stomachic as well as an effectual antispasmodic in colic and stomach pains. A powerful diaphoretic known to promote the eruptions of such minor blood diseases as measles and scarlet fever, it is infused with catnip and yarrow and the warm tea is taken every hour or two. Saffron tea is also helpful in liver disorders. Its content of vitamin B-2 is said to be the richest source known, having three times the amount of riboflavin as yeast or liver.

SAGE
Salvia officinalis

SYNONYM   Garden Sage

PART USED   The leaves.

SIGNATURE   1. In European countries, the herb grows best in mountainous sections or limestone formations, with almost a minimum of soil, thus yielding the optimum of volatile oil.

2. The soft downy hairs.

3. As in the case of hoarhound and coltsfoot, the ground herb, when pressed together, clings to itself and stays in a compact mass.

SPECIFIC USE   1. Sage directs its stimulating therapeutic action toward the liver, kidneys, and gallbladder, from which latter two organs it helps to remove gravel and stone formations. For this purpose, the herb is usually combined with others of similar but gentler nature such as dandelion and yarrow.

2. Its peculiar sharply aromatic odor and taste are long remembered when its warm infusion is drunk to remedy an irritation or tickling of the throat, a pain in the side, or a persistent nervous irritableness. It is an excellent carminative which helps expel the sharp pains caused by gas or wind and one of the best tonic-restoratives in debility of the nervous system.

3. Here is an indication of its astringent action and its cleansing and detoxifying power. Sage's ability to heal affections of the mouth and throat is well known, for its centuries-old use as a mouthwash and gargle is still recommended in many countries for a quinsy, sore throat, mouth ulcers, and inflamed tonsils. Its strong diaphoretic action flushes the catarrhal deposits from the mucous linings of the alimentary and

bronchial canals to help prevent and overcome gastric problems, colds, and pectoral disorders.

CLARY SAGE
Salvia sclarea

SYNONYMS   Clary, Clear-Eye, See Bright

PARTS USED   The seeds, leaves, herb.

SIGNATURE   1. The velvety hairs which cover the leaves and stems.

2. The herb grows best in limestone, on hills and mountains, and in other barren areas with very little soil.

3. The mucilaginous seeds.

SPECIFIC USE   1. Like garden sage, the herb has been employed to stop tickling of the throat and chest. The aromatic leaves are a warming carminative and tonic for colic, nausea, and temporary discomforts of the stomach and intestines. An infusion of the leaves soothes irritated mouth affections, cankers, and sore throat.

2. Clary is an effective remover of catarrhal sediment in the kidneys, liver, gallbladder, and bronchial organs.

3. Since early in the seventeenth century eye salves and lotions have included the seeds' mucilage. The seeds were also applied as a poultice to tumors and swellings, and the hairy leaves to slowly healing sores and ulcers, insect bites, and scratches.

ST. JOHNSWORT
Hypericum perforatum

PARTS USED   The leaves and flowering tops.

SIGNATURE   1. The leaves seem to be perforated with many

pellucid dots which are full of oil, thus its specific name, *perforatum.*

2. The bruised flowers yield a reddish, resinous juice.

SPECIFIC USE   An ointment or tincture of the flowers is most useful for skin eruptions, scratches, insect bites, general skin irritations, and wounds.

WILD SARSAPARILLA
Aralia nudicalis

SYNONYMS   False, Virginian, or American Sarsaparilla

PART USED   The root system.

SIGNATURE   The roots display a long creeping system that grows horizontal to the level of the earth.

SPECIFIC USE   The signature identifies this member of the ginseng family directly with the bloodstream. Its use as an alterative and stimulant in blood and skin ailments and in rheumatic conditions has been unparalleled. Indian herbalists recommended it to promote blood purification during pregnancy and for painless childbirth.

SASSAFRAS
Sassafras albidum, S. variifolium

SYNONYMS   Ague Tree, Saxifrax, Mitten Tree, Gumbo, Cinnamon Wood

PARTS USED   The leaves, pith, bark of root.

SIGNATURE   1. The popular name is derived from saxifrage, a rock-breaking plant known to the Romans (*saxum,* "stone," and *frangere,* "to break"). Both tree and plant seem to sprout in the clefts of rocks, as though they had broken through to display their power of shattering hard substances.

2. The principal constituent of the light pith and leaves is their mucilage.

SPECIFIC USE   1. Sassafras's diuretic and stimulating actions are most useful in kidney and blood disorders. Its gentle cleansing quality removes stone-forming gravel and similar concretions from the urinary passages. And it is still a good "blood purifier."

2. The leaves are much used in the South as a thickening agent in Creole soup and stew recipes, but it is interesting that the Choctaw Indians taught the whites the various culinary applications of this wonderful herb. In Louisiana, under the name of *gumbo filé,* the powdered sassafras leaves unite their mild, sweet fragrance and mucilaginous effect to yield a soup that has not varied much since primitive Indian times. The demulcent property of this anticatarrhal performer recommends the leaves for most internal disorders, as well as for removal of obstructions from the mucous linings. The spongy pith, once removed from the dried stems, yields an eye lotion which quickly soothes local inflammation and helps to remove irritating matter from the eye.

SAXIFRAGE
Saxifraga virginiensis, S. pennsylvanica

SYNONYMS   Rockfoil, Stonebreak

SIGNATURE   Its habitat is one of rock crevices and coarse gravelly areas.

SPECIFIC USE   The habitat suggested to early Roman physicians as well as American Indian doctors the use of this stonebreaking herb in diseases of the kidneys and bladder.

FIELD SCABIOUS
Scabiosa arvensis

LESSER SCABIOUS
Scabiosa columbaria

PART USED   The herb.

SIGNATURE   The scaly pappus of the seeds corresponds to a type of leprosy, scales, or scurf, hence the derivation of the common name Scabious from the Latin *scabere*, "to scratch."

SPECIFIC USE   The herb became a specific in leprous conditions, for itch and mange, dandruff and skin scales, to which a sponge of a strong decoction was generally applied.

SCULLCAP
Scutellaria laterifolia

SYNONYMS   Quaker Bonnet, Helmet Flower, Madweed

PART USED   The overground portion.

SIGNATURE   The generic name, *Scutellaria*, from the Latin *scutella*, "a little dish," describes the bell-shaped lid of the calyx as a cap- or helmet-like protuberance. Thus this "little dish for the head" was suggested by the early herbalists for "noises and ailments of the skull."

SPECIFIC USE   In almost constant use for over two hundred years, scullcap has been accepted as a superior tonic, nervine, and antispasmodic in all nervous disorders, sleeplessness, and headaches.

SCURVY GRASS
Cochlearia officinalis

SYNONYM   Spoonwort

PART USED   The entire herb.

SIGNATURE   1.   The herb grows profusely in stony and mountainous areas, in sandy soil, along the sea coast, and in wet places.

2.   The succulent leaves.

SPECIFIC USE   When at first this ubiquitous plant was employed as a stimulating diuretic to eliminate toxins and gravel from the kidneys and bladder and the results found highly admirable, other benefits were noticed, especially its action against the symptoms of scurvy and rheumatic complaints. Seamen prevented these distressing conditions long before vitamin C (the antiscurvy factor) was known, storing large bales of the tangy leaves aboard their ships before long sea voyages. The plants were eaten either in salads or with soup. Before the easy availability of lemons and other citrus fruits, scurvy grass was the only herb known to Captain James Cook and other seafaring men of his day that could prevent the scourge of sailors while voyaging around the world.

SELF-HEAL
Prunella vulgaris

SYNONYMS   Heal-All, Woundwort, Brunella, Sickle Wort, Carpenter's Weed

PART USED   The herb.

SIGNATURE   The flowers seen in profile resemble, it was said, a grass-cutting sickle. To herbalist William Coles, each flower consisted of a mouth and throat, and so the herb was considered an infallible remedy for "an extraordinary inflammation or swelling, as well in the mouth as throat."

SPECIFIC USE   Self-heal has been a centuries-old specific for extremely delicate sore throat and mouth irritations. The German *Bräune,* "quinsy," yields the synonym Brunella and the generic name *Prunella.* A strong decoction is used not only for an astringent-styptic gargle but also to soothe and help repair the weakened stomach and intestines during or following diarrhea, with far better results than are offered by today's proprietaries.

SENNA PODS
Cassia acutifolia, Cassia angustifolia

PART USED   The fruits.

SIGNATURE   The brown reniform or elliptical legumes were thought to resemble the human stool.

SPECIFIC USE   Senna pods have been used as a laxative for over eleven centuries and have been preferred to the leaves, since they do not contain the resin that causes griping. The pods are especially suitable in habitual constipation, the action being principally on the lower bowel.

SEPTFOIL
Potentilla tormentilla

SYNONYMS   Tormentil, Seven Leaves

PARTS USED   The roots. The entire herb.

SIGNATURE   The quite slender procumbent stems grow upon the ground, often scrambling on barren or dry soil. The herb must be gathered in late fall when the stems are completely red.

SPECIFIC USE   This is a typical needle-and-thread herb, displaying its healing qualities by staying close to the skin of the earth. Septfoil is a powerful astringent, with a potency indicated by its generic name. It imparts strength and tone to weakened muscles during an attack of dysentery, and serves as well to heal a sore throat or an ulcerated mouth, and stops hemorrhages from the nose and teeth. The herb's bitter tonic and healing properties strengthen the digestive system, for which an infusion of the summer-collected herb may be taken three or four times a day.

SHEEP SORREL
Rumex acetosella

SYNONYMS   Sour Grass, Sour Dock

PART USED   The herb.

SIGNATURE   1. It requires sandy or stony places for growth.
2. The red stems.

SPECIFIC USE   1. Its primary benefits are those of diuretic and refrigerant, which result in cleansing the urinary organs. Its antiscorbutic property has been known for centuries.
2. This little herb is still used in blood disorders, in eruptions and other skin problems. The herb also forms a cool and pleasant drink which is most useful in fevers and inflammatory disorders. Remember that sorrel means "sour," from the acidity of the leaves.

SHEPHERD'S PURSE
Capsella bursa-pastoris

SYNONYMS   Pepper and Salt, Lady's Purse

PART USED   The entire plant.

SIGNATURE   1. The herb flourishes almost year long in all parts of the world outside the tropics, and even in the arctic regions. Although the herb may be found in all kinds of soil, growing in ordinary or garden soil produces taller plants but less pungent leaves, as well as less diuretic potency and astringency.
2. The diminutive triangular seed pouches appear to be joined together like an old-fashioned leather purse.
3. The pods contain numerous tiny seeds.

SPECIFIC USE   1. This profuse grower is not only unmindful of hot or cold weather; it disregards being trampled upon for it will only rise again and persist in flourishing. Such universality would seem to indicate its high purpose: shepherd's purse is an all-purpose provider, a good food as well as medicine, and its benefits need to be better recognized.

2. The joining together of the wedge-shaped seed valves represented healing, a specific astringent and hemostatic in all kinds of hemorrhages—of the stomach, lungs, and kidneys. Only two generations ago, the herb attracted the attention of the medical world not only in the treatment of uterine hemorrhages but for its stimulating action on the uterine muscles. Its astringent effect is also required in chronic diarrhea of humans and animals. During World War I, when two widely used hemostats, ergot and goldenseal, became unavailable from European sources, they were replaced with an extract of shepherd's purse with excellent results. Its styptic qualities are easily obtained by decocting the fall-gathered herb in hot water, or simmering it in unsalted lard to yield a good healing ointment. Both preparations help to heal wounds, scratches, ulcers, and the like.

3. It is a soothing, stimulating diuretic, useful in catarrhal inflammations of the urinary organs. Not only does it increase substantially the flow of urine, it also helps to remove mucous matter from urine.

SILVER WEED
Potentilla anserina

SYNONYMS   Goose Tansy, Cramp Weed, Silver Cinquefoil

PART USED   The entire herb.

SIGNATURE   1. The plant thrives in dry, barren soil or on gravelly or sandy shores.

2. The root produces a reddish dye. The fruit resembles a dry strawberry.

SPECIFIC USE 1. An infusion of the herb has been much employed in gravel formations of the kidney passages.

2. The reddish color resulting from a decoction of the fall-collected roots recommended its use as an excellent gargle for sore throat and mouth wash for bleeding gums. Especially has the decoction been efficacious as an injection for bleeding piles, as an astringent remedy for bleedings of all kinds, internal and external, and as a general vulnerary. An infusion of the herb itself is used in painful dysmenorrhea.

SKUNK CABBAGE
Symplocarpus foetidus

SYNONYMS Meadow or Swamp Cabbage, Skunkweed, Dracontium

PART USED The roots.

SIGNATURE 1. The plant grows abundantly in swampy and wet woods.

2. The cabbage head, when cut transversely, appears to represent the human thorax.

SPECIFIC USE The roots of this herb, Thoreau's "hermit of the swamp," have been a long-respected remedy in various chest complaints. Therapeutically, they are a very active diaphoretic and expectorant in chronic bronchial and asthmatic complaints, catarrhal affections, and whooping cough. It is said that the early settlers imitated such use from their Indian teachers.

SOAPWORT
Saponaria officinalis

SYNONYMS Soaproot, Bouncing Bet

PARTS USED The roots. The herb.

SIGNATURE   The reddish-brown root of this coarse perennial system imparts in water a lather-forming property.

SPECIFIC USE   A saponin called *saporubin* is responsible for the sudsing action as well as for the herb's employment as a valuable alterative and a former substitute for sarsaparilla in gout and rheumatism. The plant's name is self-explanatory: the root's frothing ability led to its use as an all-purpose soap wash and for scouring dishes and pans. Moreover, it has been used with red clover blossoms as an excellent shampoo and a decoction will remedy skin itch and various cutaneous conditions.

SOLOMON'S SEAL
Polygonatum officinale

SYNONYM   Sealroot

PART USED   The roots.

SIGNATURE   1.   The common name was suggested by the flat round scars on the rootstock, which resemble the seal of Solomon, a six-pointed star formed by two intersecting equilateral triangles. One herb authority claims that a transverse cutting of the root reveals a resemblance to Hebrew alphabet-characters used by King Solomon "who knew the diversities of plants and the virtues of roots" and who had supposedly stamped his seal of approval upon the root in testimony of its great medicinal virtues. The generic name *Polygonatum* signifies "many-angled," indicating the knots or swellings of the jointed root, with circular scars left at intervals by the leaf stems of previous years.

2.   The mucilaginous principles of the fresh stem and root.

SPECIFIC USE   1.   Herbalists world-wide and throughout the years have recommended the roots to insure quick healing. The American Indian applied the bruised and water-warmed root as

a poultice to remove swellings. The French called it *l'herbe
de la rupture,* to heal and seal wounds.

2. The roots have also been employed for their mucilagi-
nous-healing properties. Its demulcent action is well suited in
cough syrups for pectoral complaints when painful expectoration is occasioned. Because of its mucilage and pectin contents
the root is indicated as a restorative in bowel complaints. It is
often given as a diuretic in urinary disorders; the action may be
due to the asparagine content, which is found also in marsh
mallow and asparagus.

FALSE SOLOMON'S SEAL
Smilacina racemosa

SYNONYM   Wild Spikenard

SIGNATURE AND SPECIFIC USE   The same as those of Solomon's Seal (see above).

SPEARMINT
Mentha spicata

SYNONYMS   Lady's, Garden, or Mackerel Mint

PART USED   The overground portion.

SIGNATURE   The mint prefers moist soil and is usually found
on the sides of brooks and in cool, moist situations.

SPECIFIC USE   It is a useful and effective anticolic and stimulating carminative in the usual catarrhal disturbances of the
alimentary system. Its antispasmodic and diuretic services are
indicated in strangury, gravel, and inflammatory problems of
the kidneys and bladder.

SPEEDWELL
Veronica officinalis

SYNONYM   Ground-Heele

PART USED   The herb.

SIGNATURE   1. It is found in poorly drained wastelands, but its preferred habitat is among rocks; thus the blue-flowered plant is often cultivated in rock gardens.

2. The woody stems trail on the ground and at times are almost prostrate.

3. The plant is covered with short hairs.

SPECIFIC USE   Centuries have passed since speedwell was first used in Germany for medicinal purposes. The name Ground-Heele is from the German *Grundheil,* literally "to heal" and "grind," a leprosy-like condition. In most European countries the little perennial was known as *thé d'Europe* and commonly substituted for Chinese tea, quite possibly because it helped to strengthen and fortify the body against disease.

1 & 2.   This all-purpose herb is indicated in blood and kidney disorders. It is clearly diuretic and alterative in action, serviceably cleansing the urinary organs of stone formations and removing catarrhal deposits from the bronchia.

3. The hairs indicate the plant's usefulness in all tickling sensations, internal and external. A tepid infusion, plain or syruped, is sipped to allay irritations of the throat and to remove nasal catarrh. The strong decoction is applied to skin affections, pimples, and slowly healing sores.

PRICKLY SPIKENARD
Aralia spinosa

SYNONYMS   Hercules Club, Prickly Elder

PART USED   The entire root system.

SIGNATURE   The stems and petioles are quite prickly.

This shrub, well armed with sharp spines which indicate pain throughout the body, may be considered an all-purpose remedy. (It is a member of the Ginseng, the panacea herb, family.) Its alterative accommodations were well known to the Indian medicine men, to the early settlers, and to the recent compilers of medical compendia. Its value was stressed in rheumatic, blood, and cutaneous affections and its infusion, when mixed with maple syrup or sugar, served as a stimulating diaphoretic in colds, coughs, and other pectoral affections.

SPRING BEAUTY
Claytonia virginica

PART USED   The herb.

SIGNATURE   1. It is found in moist woods and low meadows.
2. The succulent leaves.

SPECIFIC USE   Both signatures indicate the herb's use as a kidney stimulant. Its mucilaginous base has caused the entire plant, especially the rounded roots, to be used as a potherb.

SPRUCE
Picea canadensis

PART USED   The gum.

SIGNATURE   A continual supply of the exuding resinous gum appears in the ruptures or in prepared incisions in the tree bark.

SPECIFIC USE   To the North American Indian, the hardened pitch first represented the mucus secretions which needed to be ousted from the throat and chest. For this purpose a warm tea of the leaves was drunk following the use of the gum and leaves as a sweating agent and/or an inhalant for colds. It is quite likely that the medicine man, upon chewing the gum well before applying to a deep cut or sore, discovered its expectorant quality in this manner.

SPURGE
Euphorbia pilulifera

SYNONYMS   Asthma Weed, Pill-Bearing Spurge

PART USED   The overground portion.

SIGNATURE   The resinous juice yielded by the torn leaves or stem.

SPECIFIC USE   The name Spurge was taken from the Latin *expurgare*, "to purge" or "to clean." The herb was given to the asthmatic to dislodge and expel the catarrhal "juice" from the bronchial tubes and to correct chronic inflammatory conditions of the respiratory ducts.

SQUILL
Urginea maritima, U. indica

SYNONYMS   Sea Onion, White Squill

PART USED   The dried scales of the bulb.

SIGNATURE   1. The squill bulbs grow in sandy places along the sea coast or on gravelly hills.

2. The flower-stem is succulent and round; the bulb scales, mucilaginous.

3. The juicy scales appear in concentric layers, closely pressed against one another.

SPECIFIC USE   All signatures clearly denote its diuretic property. The scales were originally used for its stimulating effect upon the kidneys. Consequently, it became a standard remedy in dropsy, whether caused by a chronic kidney ailment or renal congestion prior to or resulting in cardiac impairment. For the latter condition squill was often combined with digitalis, another diuretic-cardiac stimulant. The succulent stems and mucilaginous scales led to its use, in small doses, as a stimulating expectorant to loosen the thickened phlegm from the mucous lining of the bronchia.

WHITE STONECROP
Sedum acre and varieties

SYNONYM   Live-Long

PARTS USED   The leaves and stalks.

SIGNATURE   1. The habitat—damp, sandy places, on rocks and stone walls (thus the common name).
2. The jelly-like exudation of the very juicy leaves.

SPECIFIC USE   Both signatures show the herb's affinity for liquid and stone, and thus its healing value as a quick refrigerant and diuretic-resolvent in the inflammation of and in stone removal from the kidney apparatus. It was also used in dropsy. However, the second signature should be equated with other discharges, especially of the skin and nasal passages. The mucilaginous substance has been applied to slowly healing ulcers, burns, pus-forming sores, painful warts, and other excrescences. Also, it may be used, as has the expressed exudation of Virginian stonecrop, *Sedum penthorum,* to relieve chronic nasal catarrh with comparable efficacy.

STONEROOT
Collinsonia canadensis

SYNONYMS   Horse- or Ox-Balm, Knob-Root

PART USED   The fresh roots.

SIGNATURE   1. The knobby root.

2. The plant resides in wet woods.

3. A chief ingredient is its mucilage content.

SPECIFIC USE   1. The root swellings may have first signaled the Indian herbalist to apply it to swollen wounds and sprains.

2 & 3. Its main actions, however, are those of diuretic and stimulating diaphoretic. The herb greatly improves, as the name Stoneroot implies, most calculous affections and chronic catarrhal problems of the bladder. And the mucilage yielded by this perennial exerts its benefits upon all mucous linings.

STORAX
Liquidambar orientalis, L. styraciflua

SYNONYMS   Styrax, Sweet Gum

PART USED   The balsam obtained from the inner bark and wood of the tree.

SIGNATURE   This is a pathological resinous product from the oil ducts of the injured tree part.

SPECIFIC USE   A remedy of long standing in the countries of the Mediterranean, it is of great value as an external application (in ointment form) in skin disorders, and also as a well-known stimulating expectorant, most useful in raising and discharging pathological mucous formations from the throat and bronchial tubes. The balsam is an ingredient of the popularly used Tincture Benzoin Compound.

WILD STRAWBERRY
Fragaria virginiana

GARDEN STRAWBERRY
Fragaria vesca

PARTS USED   The fruits, leaves, roots.

SIGNATURE   1. The fruits' redness.

2. The running stems or vines by which the plant covers the ground, trying to form new plants.

3. The numerous very small seeds of the fruits.

SPECIFIC USE   1 & 2. To the fruits are attributed several well justified therapeutic claims. Foremost is its power to enrich the bloodstream with its quickly assimilated major minerals—sodium, calcium, potassium, iron, sulfur, and silicon—and the associated citric and malic acids. The fruit has also been a useful tartar-removing dentifrice, its freshly expressed juice serving to remove dental discoloration by being allowed to remain on the teeth a few minutes and then rinsed off with warm water. Linnaeus, the famous Swedish botanist, first demonstrated that the berries were an excellent remedy—or a near cure—for gout and rheumatic disorders. One must also take note that the fruits are an outstanding source of vitamin C, which today is vitally needed for the prevention and treatment of scurvy.

1 & 3. Color and seeds also represented a remedy for maladies of the liver and gallbladder, for which teas of the leaves, accompanying the eating of the fruits, were taken usually without eating other foods for several days. Of greater therapeutic significance are its catarrh-removing and stone-dissolving capabilities, of great benefit to the alimentary and urinary structures. A decoction of the astringent fall-collected stems and roots soon heals a sore throat and mouth sores, and diluted with an equal part of water is a strengthening tonic for convalescents and especially for children having bowel and bladder weakness.

SUGAR CANE
Saccharum officinarum

PART USED   The expressed juice.

SIGNATURE   The mucilage and saccharine matter which is obtained from the white juicy pith of the stems.

SPECIFIC USE   In its *original* state, the cane's juice and pith are most nutritive, antiseptic, and demulcent. Medicinally, it is used in tropical and subtropical countries as a pectoral in catarrhal affections and to relieve hoarseness and tickling coughs.

SMOOTH SUMAC
Rhus glabra

STAGHORN SUMAC
Rhus typhina, R. hirta

PARTS USED   The fruits, bark, and excrescences.

SIGNATURE   1. The red fruits appear in dense clusters which resemble accumulations of pathogenic bacteria responsible for tonsillitis, diphtheria, and similar conditions. The fruits are collected late in fall.

2. A milky juice exudes from broken stems or leaf joints.

3. The small round excrescences and bark openings.

4. The velvety hairs that completely cover the tree trunk and stems.

SPECIFIC USE   1. The astringent fruits are strongly antiseptic and have been extensively used as a mouthwash and gargle for soreness and irritations of the throat, cankers, and inflamed tonsils. "Indian Lemonade," a simple, sweetened infusion of the immature berries, tends to nullify the activity of pathogenic bacteria along the alimentary and bronchial tubes. A simultaneous benefit of the tart solution occurs when it cleanses out the annoying catarrh forming along these passages, while it helps to reduce temperature in feverish conditions.

2 & 3. The hardened juice and the excrescences, which consist principally of gallic and tannic acid, are ingredients of a remarkable ointment which quickly heals cuts, scratches, and infected sores. The bark also enters an ointment formula for burns, and in decoction form is an amazingly fast hemostatic. The exuding milk is not only applied to warts and moles; it is

allowed to harden to a semi-solid state and inserted into a dental cavity.

4. The long hairs of the sumacs advise the herbalist that the tree's usable parts will greatly help to stop the vexing irritations caused by the aforementioned disorders.

Rhus hirta is an outstanding example of a common plant or tree whose fresh leaves and stems have yielded antibiotic substances of major importance. These substances inhibit *in vitro* at least forty-three microorganisms.

SUNFLOWER
Helianthus annus

SYNONYM   Marigold of Peru

PARTS USED   The seeds and leaves.

SIGNATURE   This all-purpose annual has extraordinary powers of absorbing large quantities of moisture; thus it has become a most useful instrument for drying swampy lands and damp soils.

SPECIFIC USE   The herb's usable parts have diuretic and diaphoretic action and have been employed successfully in bronchial and pulmonary affections, as in coughs and colds. The parts are simmered with boneset, yarrow, and sarsaparilla to produce a cough syrup.

TAMARACK
Larix laricina

SYNONYMS   American Larch, Hackamatack

PARTS USED   The bark. The gum.

SIGNATURE   1. This graceful tree grows in swamps and on the marshy borders of lakes and ponds.

2. The fragrant resinous exudation, which is easily separated from the bark in hot water.

SPECIFIC USE   1. The Indians called tamarack the "swamp tree" and used its various parts to cleanse the passages of harmful muck from the mucous linings. The removal of such toxins necessitated gentle diuretic and laxative activities and the bark's alterative property was to be evidenced in liver and cutaneous complaints. The Ojibwe doctor advised using the dried leaves as an inhalant and sweating plant in colds and coughs, while the bark was highly valued to produce copious expectoration in chronic bronchitis. It was also employed in inflammatory affections of the urinary organs.

2. Since earlier Indian times, the gummy exudation has been employed as a substitute for spruce gum and especially as a local remedy for skin problems, and, with the fresh leaves, as an application to burns.

TANSY
Tanacetum vulgare

SYNONYM   Yellow Buttons

PARTS USED   The early leaves and flowering tops.

SIGNATURE   1. It grows mainly in stony waste places and sandy roadsides.
2. The yellow flowers.

SPECIFIC USE   1. Its stimulating, aromatic, and diaphoretic properties make it an invaluable remedy for removing not only the sludgy catarrh from the mucous lining of the viscera but especially the stone obstructions from the urinary apparatus and the passages leading to the gallbladder.

2. Its cleansing virtues are well represented in dyspepsia and jaundice when used with other aromatics. However, tansy must be used with caution, preferably under the direction of an herbalist, and then in rather small doses.

HOLY THISTLE
Cnicus benedictus

SYNONYM   Blessed Thistle

PART USED   The overground portion.

SIGNATURE   Cruelly sharp, prickly hairs cover the leaves and flowerheads, and a thin, bristly down covers every part of the plant.

SPECIFIC USE   The name Thistle, from the Anglo-Saxon *pistel,* from *pydan,* "stab," clearly emphasizes the above characteristic. The herb is an old established remedy "for pain and stitch," from head to toe, from one side to the other, front and back, inwardly and outwardly. It was early recognized as an all-purpose herb for all maladies known to man, strengthening "all principal members of the body, as the brain, the heart, the stomach, the liver, the lungs, and the kidneys." We find herbalist Turner saying, "It is good for any ache in the body and strengthens the members of the whole body, and fastens loose sinews and weak." And herbalist Culpepper: "It helps plague sores, boils, and itch." Other reports noted its frequent recommendation for "stitches of the side," for pains arising from disorders of the liver and gallbladder, and from gouty, rheumatic conditions. (Thistle's active ingredient, cnicin, is said to be analogous to the salicin of willow and poplar, which have known and proven anti-arthritic properties.) Indian doctors employed native thistles for all pains and spasms of the stomach, and those due to female dysfunctions.

THROATWORT
Campanula trachelium

PARTS USED   The roots and herb.

SIGNATURE   The corolla was said to resemble the throat. The hair growth throughout the stem and corolla was probably of equal value as a signature.

SPECIFIC USE   The herb was believed to be good for irritations and affections of the throat. In all probability it gave proper evidence of its therapeutic ability, for it warranted the specific name *trachelium,* from the Greek *trachelos,* "neck."

WILD THYME
Thymus serpyllum

GARDEN THYME
Thymus vulgaris

SYNONYMS for Wild Thyme: Creeping Thyme, Mother of Thyme

SYNONYM for Garden Thyme: Common Thyme

PART USED   The herb.

SIGNATURE   1. Considered as a whole, the outline of the growing plant was said to correspond to the inverted shape of the chest. Note that the branches creep out from the center stem as do the thoracic bones from the spinal cord. *Serpyllum,* from the Latin *serpens,* "creeping," describes well the nature of growth of wild thyme: prostrate and spreading out on the ground, usually two to three inches in height and found in barren, sandy soil.

2. Thyme thrives in hot, dry places or between cool, damp bricks or flagstones, in the crevices of stone steps, in rock gardens. Garden thyme is a low shrubby plant and is often cultivated as a ground cover.

SPECIFIC USE   1. Thyme and its extracts have a long, respected reputation for their therapeutic action on the bronchial structure. It formed the main ingredient of the old Pertussin formula and one of two of Diatussin, a prescription product indicated, like the herb itself, in spasmodic, irritating coughs, whooping cough, and coughs due to colds.

2. Stimulant and carminative properties are indicated when-

ever there is a tendency for the catarrh to linger along the mucous linings of the alimentary, bronchial, and urinary systems. Especially from the latter area do the comfortably aromatic principles tend to remove the possible gravel deposits that may result in kidney stones. The name Thyme is taken from the Greek, meaning either "to fumigate" or "to sacrifice," in reference to the use of its fragrant, balsamic wood as incense-bearing firewood for the sacrifice altars.

TOLU
Myroxylon balsamum, Toluifera balsamum

PART USED   The balsam which results from intentional injury to the tree's trunk.

SIGNATURE   The exudations represent the principle which corrects the mucous and catarrhal discharges and the pus formations of external sores.

SPECIFIC USE   This amorphous resin is credited with antiseptic and stimulating expectorant properties that are needed in chronic catarrhal and inflammatory chest complaints. Even during the 1950s, physicians still prescribed syrup of tolu, alone or combined with other ingredients, as a reliable cough remedy.

TRAGACANTH
Astragalus gummifer and species

SYNONYM   Gum Tragacanth

PART USED   The gummy exudation which swells but does not dissolve in water.

SIGNATURE   The gelatinous mass simulates the mucous formations of throat and bronchia.

SPECIFIC USE   The gum has been much used as a demulcent, especially in pharyngitis. It also helps to suspend insoluble powders which are to be incorporated in commercially prepared throat lozenges.

TREFOIL
Oxalis acetosella

SYNONYMS   Shamrock, Wood Sorrel

PART USED   The whole herb.

SIGNATURE   1. The heart-shaped leaves.
    2. The herb is found in the cool shade, in damp woods, and next to the foundations of houses.

SPECIFIC USE   1. Such leaf structures must have attracted the attention of the early herbalists, who recommended it as food and medicine to one ailing with a heart condition. A change to a near vegetarian diet and drinking teas brewed with trefoil leaves also helped.
    2. While this is no "sure-cure," the general idea is the same: the herb directs its benefits mainly through the kidneys and bladder, then toward the bloodstream and indirectly to the heart. The cordate leaves are a good diuretic-refrigerant in most urinary problems and inflammatory diseases.

TURMERIC
Curcuma longa

PARTS USED   Rhizome and roots.

SIGNATURE   The yellow color of the flowers and the prepared rhizomes (entire root system).

SPECIFIC USE   It was formerly esteemed as a mild aromatic bitter and stimulant to the liver and as a specific in jaundice, to remove catarrhal formations and "obstructions" leading to the liver and gallbladder. The *U.S. Dispensatory* states that the oil of turmeric yields curcumen, a substance which dissolves cholestrin, a major component of bile and gallstones; it is there-fore of protective value to the gallbladder.

TURPENTINE

SYNONYMS   Resin, Oil of Turpentine

PART USED (also the SIGNATURE)   The sticky, gummy juice or exudation of pines, larches, and other coniferous trees, called resin or rosin, oleoresin, balsam, pitch, or (when the tree wood is subjected to heat) tar.

SPECIFIC USE   The exudation is used quite extensively as an in-gredient of healing ointments for open wounds and skin prob-lems, of drawing salves and plasters, as an antiseptic protective in veterinary practice, and as a stimulating counter-irritant in liniments. Internally, crude turpentine has been chiefly employed as a stimulating expectorant in cough syrups.

TURTLE-HEAD
Chelone glabra

SYNONYMS   Balmony, Snake Head, Salt-Rheum Weed

PART USED   The herb.

SIGNATURE   Its habitat is wet places.

SPECIFIC USE   Its tonic and slightly aperient qualities assist the removal of toxic sludge from the stomach and intestines that so often leads to dyspepsia and debility of the digestive tract. For that reason it is recommended in cases of indigestion, in hepatic and gallbladder complaints and inflammatory disorders.

FALSE UNICORN
Chamoelirium luteum

SYNONYMS   Helonias, Blazing Star

PART USED   The root system.

SIGNATURE   1. The plant is found in moist low grounds.

2. A color of yellow predominates—in the anthers, the yellowish brown of the rhizome's upper exterior, and the yellowish orange of the lower portion. That of the active ingredient, chamoelirin, is light yellow to yellowish red.

SPECIFIC USE   1. Its initial use as a stimulating diuretic may well have led to its being employed as a uterine tonic in amenorrhea and dysmenorrhea.

2. The herb's value in liver problems was a welcome partner to its stimulant-tonic property in genito-urinary weakness.

VALERIAN
Valeriana officinalis

SYNONYMS   Setwall, Phu

PART USED   The roots.

SIGNATURE   1. The short root-stalk has many fine-meshed merging roots and rootlets which were said to resemble the brain structure.

2. This handsome plant enjoys growing in crevices and rocky walls of gardens and damp woods.

SPECIFIC USE   1. Its properties are principally antispasmodic, nervine, and anodyne. The physician of a generation ago was well aware of valerian's outstanding influence on the cerebrospinal system and its being an easily tolerated calmative in nervousness and insomnia.

2. This signature, in connection with the first, shows that very often painful or habitual dysuria or constipation is brought on by a serious agitation or breakdown in the nervous system. Valerian's aromatic principles were also considered as a stimulant and diuretic in kidney troubles.

VANILLA
Vanilla planifolia

PART USED The full-grown, unripe fruit.

SIGNATURE This is a tall climbing epiphyte whose aerial roots fasten themselves to a nearby tree from which it receives nourishment.

SPECIFIC USE Three centuries ago Mexican physicians used much of it to flavor various dishes and found it most grateful to the digestive organs and quieting to the stomach, expelling wind and aiding the diuretic function. Equally important is its beneficial stimulation upon the brain and its direct action upon the motor nerves and spinal column.

BLUE VERVAIN
Verbena hastata

SYNONYM Wild Hyssop

PART USED The entire herb.

SIGNATURE The habitat is wet places and the sides of brooks and swamps.

SPECIFIC USE Like boneset, the herb possesses diaphoretic and expectorant qualities and is most useful in feverish colds, coughs, and pleurisy. Combined with hepatics it serves well in liver and gallbladder disorders; with diuretics, in those of the kidneys and bladder. The derivation of the name Vervain emphasizes the latter; it is from the Celtic *fer*, "drive away," and *faen*, "stone."

VIBURNUM

(High Bush Cranberry Bark, True Cramp Bark, *Viburnum opulus* var. *americanum*, Sloe, Black Haw, *V. prunifolium*)

PART USED   The bark of the stem or root.

SIGNATURE   The shrub grows in or along swamps, streams, and damp localities.

SPECIFIC USE   This herb has long been recognized as a uterine sedative and spasmodic. Dr. John King was the first to aver in writing (*American Family Physician,* 1857) that the shrub's bark acted as a uterine tonic. Dr. King had discovered that his patients had learned of the uses from the neighboring Indians, specifically as an antispasmodic in hysteria, dysmenorrhea, nervous discomforts of pregnancy, periodic cramps, and the like. The viburnums found great favor with the Ojibwe, who taught the early white settlers that the bark was to be used not only in such manner but, more important, as an effective kidney stimulant in painful or spasmodic urinary conditions.

SWEET VIOLET
Viola odorata

PARTS USED   The flowers and leaves.

SIGNATURE   Their glutinous taste.

SPECIFIC USE   The herbage and flowers of fresh violets may be included in a salad, soup, or stew. One variety, *Viola esculenta* (wild okra) is very mucilaginous and is used in the South as a thickening for soup and medications. Violets have definite mucilaginous, expectorant, and emollient properties and have been much used to relieve hoarseness and inflammation of the throat, to remove, as herbalist Gerard said, "the ruggednesse of the winde-pipe and jawes," and especially to correct bronchial disorders. It has been also recommended for those with asthmatic and sinus-catarrh conditions.

     The roots of violets are a so-called nauseating expectorant and have been known to duplicate the action of ipecac.

WAKE ROBIN
Trillium erectum

SYNONYMS   Beth or Birth Root

PART USED   The rhizome and roots.

SIGNATURE   1.   The color of the ovate fruit is reddish, that of the terminal flower yellow-pinkish to purplish red, and of the external rhizome yellowish to reddish brown.
2.   The taste of the root is quite astringent and almost bitter.

SPECIFIC USE   1.   The name Birth Root arose when the early settlers noticed their neighboring Indians using it in uterine disorders and especially as a parturient. Such use was followed by the herb's employment in the treatment of metorrhagia (uterine hemorrhage) and menorrhagia (excessively profuse menstruation), and in related disorders. Then came its successful employment in the usual forms of hemorrhages, internal and external, for bleeding from lungs and rectum.
2.   Blood color and its astringency meant also the healing of external tumors, ulcers, insect bites, and nose bleed. Bloodied stools and cases of diarrhea were soon remedied with a mild decoction of the roots.

WATERCRESS
Nasturtium officinale

SYNONYMS   Tall or Water Nasturtium, Scurvy Grass

PART USED   The entire herb.

SIGNATURE   1.   It abounds in fast-moving brooks and is cultivated in shallow water sandbeds.
2.   It is a most succulent herb.

SPECIFIC USE   These signatures indicate strongly diuretic properties. The herb's known efficacy in cleansing the kidney structure has always been associated with two allied conditions. Its considerable yield of vitamin C and other important vitamins indicates its ability to help prevent scurvy, a still too common ailment bordering on arthritis. Furthermore, this vitamin also helps to prevent hardening of the arteries by maintaining the small blood vessels in a supple condition. The combination of these easily available vitamins, enzymes, and the principal blood-fortifying minerals—iron, copper, calcium, sulfur, and manganese—greatly strengthens the bloodstream. For that reason watercress is an excellent food for enriching a near-anemic type of blood and a good remedy in most blood and skin disorders.

WHITE WALNUT
Juglans cinera

BLACK WALNUT
Juglans nigra

EUROPEAN WALNUT
Juglans regia

SYNONYMS for White Walnut: Butternut, Oilnut

PARTS USED   The leaves and inner bark of the root.

SIGNATURE   1. William Cole wrote in 1657 that walnuts "have the perfect Signature of the Head . . . The outer husk or green Covering represent the Pericanium, or outward skin of the skull. . . . The inner woody shell hath the Signature of the Skull, and the yellow skin, or Peel, that covereth the Kernell of the hard Meninga and Pia-mater, which are the thin scarfes that envelop the brain. The Kernell hath the very figure of the brain and therefore it is very profitable for the brain and resists poysons."

2. The rough gray-black fissures on the trunk bark of older trees and the astringency of the mark and leaves.

SPECIFIC USE 1. At first the nut-meats came to be a favorite prescription in mental cases and in "diseases of the head," and its oil especially good for the hair and scalp. Today their appreciable quantity of such nerve-fortifying minerals as calcium, phosphorus, magnesium, and silicon insures a functioning stability of the bloodstream and brain.

2. Because of the excessive amount of tannic acid which causes the highly astringent taste, the bark and leaves were employed during the Civil War as a fast-acting remedy for diarrhea and dysentery. A strong decoction, as a cooled external application, has been used for over a century to heal sores, ulcers, and assorted skin problems. It is also a good gargle for a sore throat, cankers, and irritations of the mouth.

WATER SOLDIER
Stratiotes aloides

SYNONYMS Water Houseleek, Water Aloe

PART USED The herb.

SIGNATURE 1. The herb is an aquatic plant whose roots are well imbedded in the mud of ditches.

2. The leaves are sword-shaped, like those of aloe (therefore the specific name), with piercing prickles on the margins.

SPECIFIC USE 1. An infusion of the leaves became a popular remedy for most kidney disorders.

2. In olden days, the herb was thought to be a reliable remedy for all wounds inflicted by most iron weapons. Later, when firearms came to the fore, the leaves became a standard application for gun-shot wounds.

WHORTLEBERRY
Vaccinium corybosum

SYNONYMS Huckleberry, Highbush or Swamp Blueberry

PART USED The leaves.

SIGNATURE 1. The shrub is usually found in swamps and wet places.

2. The fruits are quite juicy and contain many seeds.

SPECIFIC USE An astringent diuretic, it is most useful in an inflamed condition of the kidneys. Extracts of the herb have been found effective against pathogenic bacteria and laboratory test organisms.

WILLOW
Salix species

PART USED The bark of the stem.

SIGNATURE Willows grow on the banks of swamps, ponds, and wet places. In North American zones, the role of willows is as important as and exactly analogous to that of the eucalyptus of sub-tropical countries, where it flourishes in swamps or marsh-lands and absorbs and transpires huge amounts of water.

SPECIFIC USE At first the herb was considered chiefly a di-uretic in urinary disorders and as a febrifuge in feverish colds. Its use as a diuretic led to its further service in genito-urinary conditions, providing relief in ovarian pain and congestion, in nervous disturbances of the menses, and in gonorrhea and sper-matorrhea. Today, and for over 200 years, the stem-bark has provided a worthy substitute for quinine and an ever-ready source of salicin, which gave us the aspirin and salicylates that are so often prescribed for today's arthritic patients.

WINTERGREEN
Gaultheria procumbens

SYNONYMS Teaberry, Mountain Tea, Spiceberry, Checker-berry

PART USED The entire herb.

SIGNATURE   1. A low procumbent herb with long slender creeping roots (stems).

2. The red berries.

3. It requires loose, sandy, acid soil, and is generally found growing in cool woods, under the shade of evergreen trees.

SPECIFIC USE   Signatures 1 and 2 state its relationship with the bloodstream. Early in the eighteenth century, native Americans drank frequent teas of this aromatic, both as a refreshing drink and as a remedy. Since then it has been employed in the more common blood and skin disorders and especially in excessive menstrual flow and bloodied stools or urine. Signature 3 indicated its use for over a century as a diuretic in catarrh of the kidneys and bladder and in cystitis. Today the oil of wintergreen is employed as a stimulant and antirheumatic.

WITCH HAZEL
Hamamelis virginiana

SYNONYMS   Winterbloom, Striped Alder, Snapping Hazelnut

PARTS USED   The leaves, twigs, and bark of stems.

SIGNATURE   The bark is covered with transverse lenticels (breathing pores).

SPECIFIC USE   The North American Indians knew well the healing virtues of the shrub. The outward appearance of the bark, with its lenticels, suggested to their herbalists that it be applied for its astringent-antiseptic quality to the aggravated openings of the body's outer covering, the skin. The Indians used the whole herb in their sweat baths to bring quick relief from a feverish cold or catarrhal cough or cases of excessive mucous discharge. A decoction of the bark was standard treatment for all kinds of hemorrhages, for poulticing all bruises, sore muscles, and painful swellings, and as a rinse for sore gums and mouth irritations. Today we applaud its astringent property for its quick hemostatic and slightly sedative tendencies. An extract prepared by the steam distillation of the twigs is used for skin irritations, burns, and insect bites; as a cold compress for headache and sore, inflamed eyes; and as an enema for painful hemorrhoids.

WOAD
Genista tinctoria

SYNONYMS   Dyer's Broom, Greenwood

PART USED   The entire plant.

SIGNATURE   The yellow flowers.

SPECIFIC USE   Woad offers a never-failing source of yellow dyestuff and for centuries the leaves have been indicated "against obstructions of the liver and gallbladder."

WOODBINE
Ampelopsis quinquefolia

SYNONYMS   American Ivy, Virginia Creeper

PARTS USED   The leaves. The twigs and bark collected after the berries have ripened.

SIGNATURE   This shrubby, woody vine displays an extensively creeping stem.

SPECIFIC USE   The use of the parts compares favorably with sarsaparilla's, as an alterative in blood and skin disorders, and as an expectorant in bronchial complaints.

WORMSEED
Chenopodium ambroides, var. *anthelminticum*

SYNONYM   Jerusalem Oak

PART USED   The dried seeds.

SIGNATURE   The minute flowers that occur in many small clusters were thought to resemble roundworms.

SPECIFIC USE   Wormseed fruits have enjoyed a long-respected position as a very active vermifuge in the herbal and orthodox treatment of roundworms (lumbricoids), for which the herb is considered one of the best expellants.

WORMWOOD
Artemisia absinthium

SYNONYMS   Absinth, Mugwort, Mingwort

PART USED   The whole herb.

SIGNATURE   1.   The small round flower heads that terminate the stems are of a yellowish tint.
   2.   The flower heads hang downward, almost vertically.
   3.   The plant grows in dry, sandy soil.

SPECIFIC USE   1.   The color yellow was an indication that the herb was intended to remove obstructions of the liver, to give good results in bilious problems, and to treat the problem of jaundice and an impaired spleen.
   2.   The drooping or nodding flower heads were thought to represent a remedy for aches of the head and a general nervine, but especially was it found helpful against epilepsy. Even the wine vermouth comes into play, for it is a French word related to "wormwood" and vermouth became known as a wine seasoned with this and other aromatic herbs. In small doses the preparation came into prominence as a preserver of the mind, from the herb's medicinal benefits as a restorative in nervous and mental disorders.
   3.   This signature is generally placed in the category of solvents and expellants of gravel or stone in the kidney apparatus. The herb served in the past two centuries as a rather vigorous diuretic for most urinary troubles and in specific dropsical cases.

MARSH WOUNDWORT
Stachys palustris

SYNONYMS   Clown's or Downy Woundwort

PART USED   The herb.

SIGNATURE   The long oblong leaves taper to a point and are covered with a soft down.

SPECIFIC USE   The hairy leaves were used in days of old instead of lint for dressing wounds caused by sword-thrusts, bleeding cuts or a deep gash. Long before the Elizabethan era, it was known as an excellent vulnerary, either as a poultice or in ointment form, which staunched bleeding and quickly healed the wound. Modern herbalists use it for similar healing purposes.

WILD YAM
Dioscorea villosa

SYNONYMS   Colic or Rheumatism Root

PART USED   The rhizome (root stalk).

SIGNATURE   1. The twining vine-like stems which cling to and run over bushes and fences.
2. The root stalk is knotty and contorted.

SPECIFIC USE   1. Twining plants have been found valuable in blood disorders and in nervous and spasmodic conditions. It is for the latter that wild yam is a remedy. Its primary use as an antispasmodic is in the eclectic treatment of bilious colic and spasms of the bowels, kidneys, and bronchia (in asthma).
2. The tropical yam, a related spices, was hailed two decades ago as a most promising and inexpensive source of a substance called botogenin. Laboratory tests revealed that this extract gave quick relief in the treatment of rheumatoid arthritis, a painful and crippling form of that complaint. The old-time

herbalists must have had good reason to apply the synonym, Rheumatism Root, to the wild yam.

YARROW
Achillea millefolium

SYNONYMS   Milfoil, Thousand Leaf, Old Man's Pepper

PART USED   The entire herb.

SIGNATURE   1. It is an herb of profusion, a never-say-die plant that grows everywhere, in all soil conditions, in every country of the north temperate zone of Europe, Asia, and America.

2. The creeping root stocks.

3. The whole plant is somewhat covered with white-grayish silky hairs.

SPECIFIC USE   1. The finely segmented leaves of this ubiquitous profuse grower display an unusually feathery appearance which led the ancients to believe that each leaf offered one thousand subdivisions (thus the synonym) equal to a thousand uses.

To many herb-users yarrow was a near panacea for ailments of the inner organs and of the skin. Ever since its varied properties were discovered—today, they are considered principally as diaphoretic, aromatic bitter, diuretic, and tonic—the herb has seen much service in feverish colds and coughs and in eruptive disorders of children such as measles and chicken pox. It is also used to tone the system in general debility or following a lengthy illness, to correct disorders of the stomach, kidneys, liver, and uterus.

2. The root stock indicates its thorough blood-cleansing property. Yarrow contains much of the blood-fortifying minerals such as iron, calcium, potassium, sulfur, and sodium, corresponding chlorides, nitrates, and phosphates, and two peculiar substances called achillein and achilleic acid. The former extract

not only has served as an effective hemostatic, to reliably and quickly reduce the clotting time of blood, but recently has been mentioned as an anti-cancer agent.

3. The hairs here indicate external irritations. A mild decoction of the entire plant is used as an astringent mouth rinse or gargle, as a vaginal wash for leucorrhea, and as an enema for hemorrhoids. A strong decoction restores healing to cuts and torn skin, indolent ulcers. This solution was extensively used by the Indians as an application to burns. And today the herb still finds a place in a healing ointment highly valued by Scotch Highlanders.

YERBA SANTA
Eriodictyon californicum, E. glutinosum

SYNONYMS   Consumptive's Weed, Gum Bush, Tar Weed

SIGNATURE   The resinous, varnish-like substance which coats the stem and the surfaces of the thick leaves.

SPECIFIC USE   The herb is a strongly stimulating, balsamic expectorant and has been much employed in bronchial and laryngeal troubles and in chronic catarrhal situations.

YUCCA
Yucca filamentosa

SYNONYMS   Adam's Needle, Spanish Bayonet, Soap Weed

PARTS USED   The leaves and root.

SIGNATURE   1. The scaly trunk. The sword-shaped, sharply-spined leaves. The fibrous peeling of the leaves' margins.

2. The soap suds that emerge from a brief shaking of the roots in water.

SPECIFIC USE   The leaf powder has proven to be a rich large-scale source of the steroid sarsapogenin, a potential cortisone precursor. The latter drug is well known in medical circles for its applications in many skin disorders. Yucca roots were, and still are, known to our Southwest Indians for their cleansing and detergent properties. The natives still employ the roots as a wash for externally-caused skin disorders, eruptions, and for slowly healing ulcers. The saponin component that is here extracted via the sudsing does not have the characteristic acrid taste of other saponins nor does it provoke sneezing.

NOT RECOMMENDED

The following plants are potentially poisonous and dangerous and therefore are expressly mentioned here:

False Acacia or Locust Tree, *Robinia pseudo-acacia*
Baneberry (White, *Actaea alba;* Red, *Actaea rubra*)
Bittersweet, *Solanum dulcamara*
False Bittersweet, *Celastrus scandens*
Buttercup, *Ranunculus* species
Buttonbush, *Cephalanthus occidentalis*
Black Root, *Leptandra virginica*
Dogbane, *Apocynum* species
Green Hellebore, *Veratrum viride*
Water Hemlock, *Cicuta maculata*
Spotted Hemlock or Cowbane, *Conium maculatum*
Mandrake, *Podophyllum peltatum*
Mountain Laurel, *Kalmia latifolia*
Stramonium, *Datura stramonium*

III

Herbal
Remedies

PREPARATION OF HERB TEAS, DECOCTIONS, AND SYRUPS

Use the following principles as a guide in preparing herb remedies.

1. All herbs must be *dried* and used whole, cut in small pieces, or finely ground.

The ingredients must be approximately uniform in size.

"Parts" may mean amounts in teaspoonsful, tablespoonsful, ounces, or handsful.

In most cases, herbs of one category may be used in equal parts and substituted for each other. For example, the buchu or cranberry leaves of a diuretic remedy may be replaced with *equal* portions of blueberry, dog-grass, horsetail, or other kidney stimulators.

2. The usual dose of single leaves and seeds is a teaspoonful steeped in a cup of hot water.

The dose: One strained cupful 3–4 times a day. *Sip slowly* and mix the liquid well with the saliva before swallowing.

A few exceptions: Purple loosestrife, 2 tablespoonsful boiled in a pint of hot water and 2 ounces of cooled liquid taken 4–5 times a day. An ounce of septfoil boiled in a pint of hot water and a wineglass dose taken every 3–4 hours. Of celandine ¼–½ teaspoonful is steeped in a cup of hot water and drunk cold morning and night.

When using several herbs, mix well and take an "average" dose (teaspoonful or tablespoonful).

The procedure: Stir 25–30 times a teaspoonful in a cup of freshly boiled water for 20–25 minutes. Cover with saucer. Stir the mixture a few times and strain. Teas of aromatics such as mints, catnip, and savory seeds are generally drunk warm to tepid and therefore are steeped 7–20 minutes. *Sip the tea slowly.* Mix the liquid well with the saliva before swallowing.

3. The usual dose of barks and roots is a tablespoonful

boiled (decocted) in a quart of hot water for a half hour, or down to half quantity (pint). The dose is ½ cupful, diluted with water, 3 times a day. Exceptions: Black cohosh, ½ teaspoonful steeped in a cup of hot water, drunk cold 3 times a day. Two tablespoonsful of oak bark boiled in a quart of hot water and a wineglass taken every hour as needed. Simmer a tablespoonful of pond lily root in 1½ pints of hot water down to a pint and drink cold one ounce 4 times a day.

The procedure: Decoct (boil) a heaping tablespoonful in a quart of hot water down to half quantity of liquid; or the decocting may last about a half hour. Use a stainless steel, porcelain, or glass (but not an aluminum) utensil. Keep the lid on at all times. Allow to cool and strain. Mix together a tablespoonful to ½ cupful of decoction in cold water and drink one such cupful 3–4 times a day. (Or the strained liquid may be divided in equal amounts, each dose taken as directed.) The dose will depend on the herb or herb mixture and on the particular circumstance for which the herbs are intended.

4. Of mixed herbs (leaves or seeds and roots) a heaping teaspoonful is gently simmered in 1½ cups for 5–7 minutes. When cool, the solution is stirred, strained, and taken, in equally divided doses, diluted in ½ cup tepid water, every 4–5 hours.

5. General principles for an herb mixture:

1 part stimulant or activator: as diuretic—pipsissewa, juniper, parsley, watercress, asparagus leaves and root; as diaphoretic—boneset, yarrow, verbena.

1 part aromatic: mints, fennel, catnip, marjoram, thyme, sassafras bark.

1 part demulcent: mallow, marsh mallow, hollyhock, sassafras leaves, Irish moss, elm.

The dose for children: Unless otherwise stated the general rule is to give children a smaller dose than that suggested for adults. The following table may be used as a guide for children's doses:

5–8   years   ⅙ to ⅓ of adult dose
8–12 years   ⅓ to ½ of adult dose
12–15 years   ½ to ⅔ of adult dose

Notes: To gain the greater benefit of the therapeutic values and efficacy of our herbal friends, the preparation, whether decoction (boiled) or infusion (steeped), is best taken on a near, if not completely, empty stomach. Thus, for best results, it is recommended to take the herbal remedies only if the diet has been limited to fruits and vegetables or if the herb-taker has not eaten for at least 5 hours. One frequently finds in herbal literature that herb teas are to be taken one hour before meals and at bedtime.

When an herb tea infusion is in order, prepare a *fresh* cupful for each dose. This does not apply to the decoction, which has been prepared to yield a concentrate.

Prepare an infusion in a porcelain cup and always cover with a saucer. Prepare a decoction in utensils of pyrex glass, enamel, or steelware. Avoid the use of aluminum.

Drink an herb tea not hot but lukewarm to tepid. An iced tea is not recommended since it is therapeutically inert. Hot and cold liquids often cause harm to the food digesting enzymes.

Sip the herb liquid *slowly,* a little at a time, a teaspoonful to a tablespoonful, and swish it around in the mouth. This will insure not only its mixing better with the ptyalin, the enzyme found in the saliva, but subsequent rapid assimilation into the bloodstream.

Try to drink an herb tea without any sweetening. If necessary, use a little honey or raw brown sugar. Keep the use of white sugar and saccharin at a minimum; if possible, *do not use at all*.

If a decoction is to be kept for the next day, refrigerate it or store in a cool place. Avoid the use of a preservative such as sodium benzoate which, like the original benzoic acid, may cause great irritation and disturbance to the stomach.

Included among herbs which should not be taken at all in

infusions are: poke, rue, senna, and other laxative-purgatives; arbor vitae (yellow cedar), elder leaves, tansy, nightshade (bittersweet); and such harsh spices as pepper, ginger, and mustard.

To prepare a syrup, *simmer* or gently decoct the herbs in the required amount of hot water for about one half hour. Stir, strain, and allow to cool. Add 2 pounds of sugar or a cup of thick honey to each pint of liquid and simmer 20–30 minutes. The dose of each syrup will depend upon the purpose for which it was intended. Cough syrups are taken in 1–2 teaspoonful doses every hour or two or as needed, blood and kidney remedies in tablespoonful doses.

THE REMEDIES

These remedies are not intended as overnight "sure cures" and cannot replace the family doctor. Herbs do not work wonders or miracles. And remember that it often takes much longer to achieve full health than the duration of one's illness. Other steps toward health besides the herbs are partial or total abstinence from food for one or several days, complete bed-rest and early to sleep, and a change to natural foods when well. Give the body an opportunity to heal itself.

AMENORRHEA
Mix equal parts of Motherwort, Smartweed, early Tansy, Skunk Cabbage, Valerian, and Pennyroyal. (In the absence of the latter two herbs, Sage and Ginger may be included, but only ¼ part of each.) Simmer 2 tsp. for 15 minutes in a pint of hot water. Take a warm cupful every 3–4 hours.

ANTACID
1. Mix equal parts of Anise, Catnip, Chamomile, Fennel, Mint, and Linden. Steep a tsp. in a cup of hot water. Drink warm 3 or 4 times a day or as needed.
2. Mix equal parts of Mint, Pennyroyal, Raspberry, Marjoram, and Catnip. Prepare as above.
3. Mix equal parts of Anise, Fennel (and/or Caraway and Dill), Catnip, and Mint. Steep a tsp. in hot water for 10 minutes. This tea is especially useful in overcoming colic in infants and the aged. For the

adults and children the dose is the entire cupful sipped slowly every hour or as often as needed. For infants, re-strain 2 oz. through absorbent cotton into a 4-ounce nursing bottle and add 2 oz. water, so that the infusion may be taken via the nipple; or the baby may prefer teaspoonful doses.

4. Mix equal parts of Mint, Valerian, Chamomile, and Catnip. Steep a tsp. in a cup of hot water 10–15 minutes. Prepare and drink a warm tea every 2 or 3 hours. For infants, prepare as indicated in #3.

ANTICOLIC See #3 and #4 of ANTACID remedies.

ANTIRHEUMATIC
REMEDY See BLOOD PURIFIER.

ANTISPASMODIC
REMEDY See CRAMP (SPASM) REMEDY.

APPETITE See STOMACHIC.

ASTHMA 1. Mix equal parts of Lobelia, Coltsfoot, Rosemary, Mullein, and Thyme.

2. Mix equal parts of Lobelia, Boneset, Valerian, Mallow, Thyme, and Wild Cherry. See COUGH #3.

Herb tea: Steep a tsp. in a cup of hot water. Add 1 or 2 drops of spirits of peppermint to each cupful. Drink tepid 3 or 4 times a day.

Syrup: Simmer a tbsp. of mixed herbs in a quart of hot water (approximately) down to half quantity. Allow to cool. To the strained solution, add 2 lbs. of brown sugar or honey (enough to make a syrup) to the pint of liquid and simmer another 15–20 minutes. When cold, add ⅔ tsp. of spirits of peppermint to the finished product. Shake well before using. The dose is 1 or 2 teaspoonsful sipped slowly as often as needed.

ASTRINGENT Mix 3 parts of Oak bark and one each of Wild Geranium root, Sumac berries and Cinquefoil (and/or equal parts of Oak, Sweet Fern, and Witch Hazel). Boil vigorously for 20 minutes one heaping tbsp. of the herbs in a quart of hot water. When cool, stir and strain.

Internally: Use ⅓–½ cup as a dose for diarrhea, etc. As a gargle use as is or diluted with a little warm water.

Externally: Apply the decoction undiluted to cuts, sores, or minor skin diseases. To use the solution (strained) as an enema for hemorrhoids or as a vaginal douche, dilute the preparation with an equal amount of tepid water before using.

Other astringent herbs which may be used: Sumac (fruits or bark), Cinquefoil, Septfoil, Gold Thread, Plantain, Life Everlasting, Wild Geranium, Water Lily root, Goldenrod, Self-Heal, Wild Indigo, Bayberry (bark), and Sweet Fern.

These herbs enter into the preparation of gargles, skin lotions and ointments, diarrhea aids, and enemas.

BATH SPECIES

Mix together 1 ounce each of Peppermint, Chamomile, Thyme, Sage, and Rosemary. Moisten the herbs with 5 oz. of (ethyl) rubbing alcohol and permit the alcohol to evaporate. Enclose the herbs in linen and allow to soak in the bath.

BLOOD PRESSURE (HIGH)

Mix equal parts of Chamomile, Elder, Mint, and Tag Alder. Steep a tsp. in a cup of hot water for 10 minutes. Drink warm 3 or 4 times a day. It is best to eat most sparingly for several days and rest in bed during that time.

Dose: Simmer gently 1 oz. in a pint of hot water for 20 minutes. Drink tepid half cupful 3 times a day.

BLOOD PURIFIER (OR BODY CONDITIONER)

1. Mix equal parts of Burdock, Yellow Dock, Dandelion, Sassafras, and Sarsaparilla (or Spikenard). To yield an "antirheumatic" remedy, add Birch Bark. Decoct 2 tbsp. in a quart of hot water down to half quantity. Take cold ½ cupful (diluted with water) 4 times a day.

2. Mix equal parts of Burdock, Dandelion, Sarsaparilla, Black Alder, and Violet or Red Clover. Prepare as indicated above.

3. Mix equal parts of Burdock, Queen of the Meadow, Yellow Dock, Barberry, and Black Alder.

(Good for eczema, boils, and skin disorders.) Boil 1
oz. of each in 1½ quarts of hot water down to half
quantity. Drink cold ½ cupful 4 times a day.
4. Mix equal parts of Thyme, Blueberry, Dandelion root, Burdock root, Watercress, and Sassafras.
Steep a tsp. in a cup of hot water. Drink cold 4 times
a day.

BRUISES
See LINIMENT.

CANKER
1. Boil ½ tbsp. each of Gold Thread and Cinquefoil (or Septfoil) in a pint of hot water down to half
quantity. Strain. Dissolve 3 tsp. of borax. Use tepid-
warm or cold as a mouthwash, or as an application to
the affected area.
2. Use (do not mix) equal parts of Gold Thread,
Sumac berries, and Sage. (In the absence of either of
the latter two, use Oak and/or Cinquefoil.) Boil 1
tbsp. of the Gold Thread and Sumac in a quart of hot
water for ½ hour. Add the Sage and simmer another
½ hour. Strain and use tepid-warm.

CARMINATIVE
See Juniper. Use ANTACID remedies.

COLD
1. Mix equal parts of Yarrow, Boneset, Mint, Catnip, Verbena, and Hoarhound, and ½ part of Sage.
Stir a heaping tsp. in cup of hot water. Cover 8–10
minutes. Drink a cupful every 2–3 hours. For children: a wineglassful.
2. See the DIAPHORETIC remedies.
Mix equal parts of Elder, Catnip, Boneset, and Peppermint, and ½ part of Sage. A tsp. of the mixture
steeped in a cup of hot water should be taken warm
4 times a day, or every hour, to produce perspiration.
To prepare a cough syrup, simmer a heaping tbsp.
of the herbs (plus one part each of Coltsfoot and
Mallow, and ½ part of Irish Moss) in a quart of hot
water for 20 minutes. When cool, strain and add the
required amount of sugar or honey. Sip slowly a
wineglassful every 2–3 hours or as required.

COLIC
Mix equal parts of Anise, Dill, Catnip, Chamomile,
Mint, and Fennel. (Or use any three.) Steep a level
tsp. in a cup of hot water for 8–10 minutes. The

adult dose is a cupful every hour, sipped slowly. For
infants, dilute with an equal portion of tepid water.
Strain carefully through absorbent cotton into a 4 oz.
nursing bottle. Give between feedings or as needed.
(See ANTACID.)

COUGH,
DUE TO COLDS

1. Mix together ½ tsp. Anise, Thyme, Boneset, and
Mallow, and two of Mullein. Simmer in 1½ cups
of hot water for 15 minutes. Allow to cool and strain.
Add the required amount of sugar or honey. Take a
tbsp. every hour or as needed. Sip slowly. (See Life
Everlasting.)

2. Mix together 3 parts of Boneset and one each of
Hoarhound, Coltsfoot, Chestnut, Irish Moss (or
Quince seeds), and Peppermint. Simmer 2 tbsp. in a
quart of hot water to yield ½ quantity (1 pint). Add
the honey or sugar. Sip slowly ½ tbsp. every hour as
required.

3. For bronchial or asthmatic spasms: Mix one
part each of Thyme, Comfrey, and Elecampane, and
½ part of Lobelia and Mallow. Prepare as in #2.
Add 1–2 drops of spirits of peppermint to each dose
before taking.

4. Bronchial cough: Mix one part each of Hoarhound, Licorice, Mallow, Comfrey, Verbena, and
Buckbean, and ½ part each of Irish Moss and Lobelia. (In the absence of any of the former six, Anise,
Wild Cherry, Boneset, Coltsfoot, Mullein, and Valerian may be considered. Prepare a syrup as directed
under #2. Add ½ tsp. of spirits of peppermint to
each pint of the finished product.

5. Child's syrup: Use equal parts of Anise, Irish
Moss, Chestnut, Thyme, Mullein, Mallow, and
Spearmint. Prepare as indicated under #2. The dose
is 1–2 tsp. every two hours.

6. Cough syrup: To each cupful of the resultant
liquid of #3 remedy under Stomachic, add half a cup
of brown sugar or honey. Sip slowly one tbsp. every
hour or as required.

7. Cough remedy: Mix a tbsp. of Life Everlasting
and 2 tsp. each of Anise seed and Thyme. Simmer a
tbsp. in 3 cups of hot water for 10 minutes. When

cold, strain and add enough brown sugar or honey to make a syrup. Take a tbsp. every 2 hours or as needed.

8. Whooping cough: Add half tsp. each of Chestnut, Elm, and Thyme to a cup of hot water. Cover until cold. Half cupful every 2–3 hours or as needed to relieve the cough. (See also COLD and DIAPHORETIC.)

CRAMP OR SPASM REMEDY

To a quart of previously warmed wine, add 1 oz. Cramp Bark (*Viburnum opulus* var. *americanum*), ½ oz. Scullcap, ½ oz. Skunk Cabbage, and 1 tsp. each of Cloves and Cinnamon. Keep in a warm area for 24 hours. Take a tbsp. in warm water 3 or 4 times a day. Or a tsp. of the herb mixture may be steeped in hot water 15 minutes, and drunk warm every 2–3 hours as needed.

CYSTITIS

Mix one part each of Cleavers, Bearberry, Dog-Grass, and half each of Catnip (or Mint), Mallow, and Sassafras. Simmer 2 tbsp. in a quart of hot water for 20 minutes. Allow to cool, and strain. Drink ½ cupful doses every 2–3 hours.

DANDRUFF (HAIR WASH)

Five parts of Soap Tree Bark (obtainable at an herbalist's shop) or 5 parts Red Clover blossoms and Soapwort (*Saponaria*) combined, 2 parts each of Quassia and Sage, and 1 each of Rosemary and Nettle. (In the absence of Sage or Rosemary, use Wormwood, Southernwood, Walnut leaves, and/or Birch leaves.) Boil a level tbsp. in a pint of hot water for 5–6 minutes. Strain and use the liquid warm-tepid as a shampoo. Massage the scalp vigorously, dry the hair, and then brush thoroughly. Do this twice a week.

DENTAL POULTICE, FOR TOOTHACHE

Mix one part of Catnip and Hops (or Summer Savory), and 2 of Sassafras. Place ½ to 1 tsp. in a piece of muslin cloth, dip in hot water for a few seconds, and apply the poultice to the affected area. Do this every ½–1 hour or as required.

DIAPHORETIC REMEDY

1. Mix equal parts of Linden flowers, Elder flowers, and Boneset. Steep a heaping tsp. in a cup of hot water. Drink warm every 1 or 2 hours.

2. Mix equal parts of Verbena, Sage, Boneset, Mint, Catnip, and Chamomile. Steep a heaping tsp. in a cup of hot water. Drink warm every 1 or 2 hours to produce sweating.

To make a syrup add enough brown sugar or honey. Drink a tbsp. cold every 2 or 3 hours, or as needed.

DIARRHEA

1. Mix equal parts of Wild Geranium, Blackberry, Oak, and Cinquefoil. Boil vigorously for 30–40 minutes ½ cupful of the herbs in 1½ quarts of hot water. Strain and add ½ tsp. each of Cloves and Ginger (or Cinnamon). Cover ½ hour. Take warm, a half cupful every hour or after each bowel movement.

2. Wild Geranium, Oak, Sumac, Sweet Fern, and Shepherd's Purse. Prepare as above.

3. See GARGLE #4.

While this condition persists, *do not eat*. Sip only enough water to satisfy thirst. Wait one full day *after* all is well before taking food.

DOUCHE

See ASTRINGENT.

DYSPEPSIA
(OR GASTRITIS)

1. Mix equal parts of Buckbean, Yarrow, Gentian, Sassafras, Sweet Flag, and Mint (also other aromatics or seasoning herbs). Simmer a tbsp. in a quart of hot water for 10 minutes. Allow to rest another 20 minutes and strain. Take tepid-warm ⅓ cupful every 3–4 hours as needed. Always take with, or dilute with, warm water.

2. Mix equal parts of Buckbean, Mallow, Sage, and Sweet Flag; Boneset and Mint may be added. Steep a tsp. in a cup of hot water ½ hour. Dilute a wineglassful with ½ cup warm water and take this 4 times a day. (Also for torpid liver.)

EARACHE
REMEDY

Place dried Mullein flowers in a cup and cover with olive or other vegetable oil. The oil mixture may be placed in direct sunlight for several days or gently warmed (indoors) for 4 or 5 hours. Each day stir the mixture. Strain. Place 3–4 drops in the ear 4–5 times a day.

ENEMA

1. Mix 1 part of Flaxseed and Chamomile and 2 of Marsh Mallow (or Mallow) leaves. Steep 2 tsp. in

a cup of hot water. Strain when tepid. Inject 3–4 times a day.

2. A decoction suitable as an injection for painful piles may be prepared by boiling 1 heaping tsp. each of Sweet Fern, Self-Heal, and Mullein in 1½ pints of hot water for ½ hour. Strain and use tepid to cool 3–4 times a day.

3. See ASTRINGENT.

EYE LOTION

Mix together ⅛ tsp. each of Chamomile, Fennel, and Eyebright. In the absence of the latter herb, use a pinch of ground Spanish Saffron or Marigold (Calendula) flowers or ⅛ tsp. Yellow Loosestrife. Steep the herbs in a cup of hot water 30 minutes. Stir and strain carefully through absorbent cotton. Allow to cool. Use in either an eye cup or a dropper every 3–4 hours. This solution may also be diluted with ⅓ amount of camphor water (prepared by soaking a small piece of pure camphor in warm distilled water for a few hours). Refrigerate the solution. To provide relief in hay fever, stir well a tsp. of Rose petals in a cup of the above steeping warm solution, and, when cool, stir and strain through absorbent cotton or filter through filter paper. Place a drop or two in each eye 4 to 5 times a day. Even a simple infusion of a tsp. of the Rose petals will be good for hay fever, for it has been proven to be almost as effective in controlling eye and nose symptoms as the druggist's Estivin, which is a "processed infusion of Rose petals."

FEVER (OR COLD)

Mix equal parts of Yarrow, Boneset, Catnip, Mint, Sage, and Verbena. Add also or substitute with Linden, Elder flowers, Pennyroyal, and Hoarhound. Steep a heaping tsp. in a cup of hot water for 8–10 minutes. Drink warm every 3–4 hours. If profuse sweating is desired, take a cupful every hour until the desired effects result. (See COLD and DIAPHORETIC.)

FOMENTATION

See POULTICE #2.

GARGLE (OR MOUTH WASH)

1. Mix equal portions of Sage and Sumac, and ¼ of Gold Thread and Cinnamon (or Cloves). In the

absence of the former two, use Wild Geranium, Oak,
Bayberry, and/or Rosemary. Simmer slowly a tbsp.
in a quart of hot water for 30 minutes or down to ⅔
the amount. Stir and strain. Gargle warm every
hour. Store balance in refrigerator. When needed,
reheat but do not boil.

2. Mix 1 part each of Life Everlasting, Cinquefoil,
and Sumac. Decoct 2 tbsp. in a pint of hot water for
10 minutes. Gargle as is or dilute with a little warm
water every ½ hour. (A cupful may be taken cold in
cases of diarrhea or summer complaints.) (See
SORE THROAT remedy.)

3. Mix equal parts of Sumac berries, Wild Indigo,
and Bayberry bark or fruits. Decoct 1 tbsp. in 1½
pints of hot water down to one. Allow to cool, and
use undiluted.

4. Gargle (or diarrhea) remedy: Mix equal parts
of Wild Geranium, Oak bark, Sumac berries, and
Sweet Fern. Boil 3 tsp. in a pint of hot water for
20 minutes. Gargle every hour. For diarrhea, drink
cold ½ cupful 4 times a day or as often as required.
(Children—a wineglassful.)

GASTRITIS   See DYSPEPSIA.

HAIR TONIC   1. Mix 1 oz. each of Rosemary and Peppergrass, 2
oz. each of Nettle and Sage. Place the finely ground
herbs in a pint of 90% alcohol for 4–5 days. Stir,
strain, and add 1 oz. each of olive and castor oils.
Slowly add enough water to cause a slight turbidity.
(See DANDRUFF.)

2. Cover ½ cup of the fruits with alcohol for one
week. To this, add one tbsp. each of Sage and Rosemary, add another ½ cupful of alcohol and allow to
stand another week. Stir occasionally. Strain and add
to the solution an equal amount of water. To each 8
oz. add 5 tsp. each castor and olive oils. Shake well
before using.

INSECT   1. Place a cup of dried Pennyroyal and Tansy
REPELLANT   flowerheads, Wormwood, Lavender, and Mints in a
pint of previously warmed alcohol (90–99%). Allow
to digest one week, and shake the bottle once daily.

2. Moth preventative: Mix equal parts of Tansy flowers, Rosemary, Pennyroyal, Lavender, and Lemon peel. Place a heaping tsp. in a small muslin bag. (See LINIMENT.)

KIDNEY STIMULANT

1. Mix 4 parts Bearberry (or Blueberry), Buchu (obtainable at a pharmacy or herb shop), Dog-Grass, Cleavers, and Mallow, 3 parts of Sassafras, Prince's Pine, and Fennel, and 1 part of Catnip, Corn silk, and Spearmint. Juniper or Horsetail may be substituted (1 part) for any of the latter three. Steep a tsp. in a cup of hot water until cold. Drink a cupful 3 or 4 times a day.

2. Mix one or equal parts of Trailing Arbutus, Burdock, Wild Carrot root, and Sassafras and 2 parts of Mallow and Dog-Grass. Simmer a tbsp. in a quart of hot water for 30 minutes. Drink tepid-cool ½ cupful, diluted with an equal portion of water, 4 times a day.

3. Mix equal parts of Prince's Pine, Bearberry (or Blueberry), Mallow, Catnip, and Dog-Grass. A tsp. to a cup of hot water. Drink cold 4 times a day.

4. Steep ½ tsp. each of Wild Carrot seeds, Bearberry, or Trailing Arbutus, and Catnip (or Mint), and 3–4 crushed Juniper berries in a cup of hot water for 10 minutes. Drink warm every 2 hours or as required.

LAXATIVE

Not recommended. Proprietary medicines should be avoided. Most of them contain harsh ingredients which may irritate the alimentary system. Often one or two days of abstinence from *all* foods—plus bed-rest—will help the system rehabilitate itself, and a complete change-over to uncooked and unprocessed fruits and vegetables greatly reactivates the bowels. Soft foods tend to harden the stools and cause constipation while raw, hard foods soften them.

LINIMENT

1. To 8 oz. of warm cider vinegar, add a level tbsp. Arbor Vitae, Wormwood, cut Cayenne (red) Pepper and Tansy flowering tops and leaves. Shake well and place on a warm radiator or other source of gentle heat for an hour. Allow to cool, strain, and add an

equal amount of spirits of turpentine in which has been dissolved ½ oz. of pure camphor. Before applying liniment, warm the affected area with warm (not hot) wet packs. For best results, gently rub in a small quantity of the liniment twice an hour for 2 or 3 hours and apply a hot water bottle or a warm, near-dry wet pack, or cover with heavy flannel.

2. Use ½ oz. each of Tansy, Wormwood, Sage, Sweet Flag, ⅛ oz. each of Wild Ginger and Cloves. Digest the herbs for two hours via moderate heat in a quart of vinegar, and keep the mixture in a tight bottle for 2 weeks. Shake the bottle occasionally. To the strained liquid add ¼ oz. camphor previously dissolved in a little rubbing alcohol. This preparation is most useful for insect bites, wounds, sprains, etc.

LIVER DISORDER

1. Mix equal parts of Dandelion, Mallow, Sweet Flag, and Fennel, and ¼ part of Celandine. Simmer a tbsp. in a quart of hot water for 30 minutes. Allow to cool. Take ½ cupful diluted with an equal portion of water 3–4 times a day.

2. Mix a tbsp. Dandelion leaves and a tsp. each Barberry, Anise, Fennel, and Mallow (or Flaxseed or Elm). Simmer a heaping tbsp. in 1½ pints of hot water for ½ hour. Take ½ cupful 3–4 times a day. (In cases of a catarrhal condition, include 1 part of Yarrow.)

3. (a) Sluggish liver: Mix 2 ounces of Dandelion leaves with ½ ounce each of Anise, Fennel, and Flaxseed (one tsp. of Celandine may be added). Simmer for 15 minutes ⅓ of the mixture in a pint of hot water, cover, and let stand a half hour. The dose is a cupful morning and night.

(b) Mix equal parts of Yarrow, Boneset, Dandelion (leaves), Chamomile or Mint, and Mallow, and ½ part of Celandine. Steep 1 tsp. in a cup of hot water 30 minutes. Drink cold 3 times a day.

MEASLES

Stir well ½ tsp. each of Yarrow and Catnip (or Elder flowers or Marjoram) and ⅛ tsp. (or a big pinch) of Spanish Saffron or Marigold flowers in a cup of hot water. Take the strained solution every 2 hours. This remedy is equally suitable for chicken pox and similar eruptive conditions, fevers, etc.

**NERVINE
(NERVE TONIC)**

1. Mix 2 parts each of Lady's Slipper, Catnip, Scullcap, and Chamomile with 1 each of Valerian and Skunk Cabbage. Steep a tsp. in a cup of hot water for 6–8 minutes. Drink half a cupful warm every 4 hours, or 3 times a day and at bedtime.

2. Mix 2 parts each of Valerian, Scullcap, and Lady's Slipper, and 1 each of Rosemary, Celery seed, and Catnip. Prepare as above.

3. Mix 2 parts of Scullcap, Chamomile, Catnip, and 1 each of Sage and Motherwort. Prepare as above.

4. Mix equal parts of Chamomile, Marjoram, Catnip, and Mint. Steep a tsp. in a cup of hot water 6–8 minutes. Drink warm, a cupful 4 times a day.

5. Nervous headache: (a) Mix 1 part Celery seed, 2 each of Catnip and Chamomile, 3 of Scullcap (latter three herbs are finely ground). (One part of Rosemary or Marjoram may replace Catnip or Chamomile.) Steep a tsp. in a cup of hot water. Drink warm every 4 hours.

(b) Nervous headache: Mix equal parts of Peppermint, Sage, and Scullcap. A tsp. to a cup of hot water. Drink tepid every 2 hours or as needed.

(c) Headache remedy: Mix a tsp. each of Sage, Catnip, Scullcap or Verbena, and ½ tsp. of Lady's Slipper. Steep a tsp. in a cup of hot water. Drink tepid every 2–3 hours.

Nerve-tone remedy: Three parts of Scullcap, 2 of Catnip, and one of Celery seed. Steep a heaping tsp. in a cup of hot water for 20 minutes. Drink warm to tepid 4 times a day.

6. "Change of Life": Mix one part of Gentian, Chamomile, Verbena, Motherwort, Scullcap, and Hops (or Valerian). Steep a tsp. in a cup of hot water. Drink warm ½ cupful, 3 times a day and at bedtime. (Replace any missing herb with any other found in other remedies of this group.)

OINTMENT See SKIN OINTMENT.

PILES See ENEMA and ASTRINGENT.

PLEURISY

1. Mix equal parts of Milkweed root, Verbena, Mallow (or Hollyhock), Yarrow, Sage, and Sweet Flag (or Wild Ginger). Simmer 2 tbsp. in a quart of hot water down to half the amount. Strain and add a tsp. of spirits of peppermint and 8 oz. honey or sugar. The dose is a tbsp. every 3 hours as needed.

2. Mix 4 parts of Milkweed, 2 each of Elder flowers, Mint, Boneset, Elacampane, and Mallow, and one of Irish Moss. Simmer 2 heaping tsp. in 1½ pints of hot water for 15–20 minutes and let stand another 30 minutes. Drink ½ cupful every 3–4 hours as needed. Sweeten if necessary.

POULTICE

1. Mix equal parts of Chamomile, Mallow, Mullein, and Sweet Clover. Place in suitable cloth and soak in hot water for 2–3 minutes. Apply as a poultice, over which is placed a hot water bottle.

2. "Foment Species": Mix 4 parts each of Lavender and Chamomile, 1 of Thyme, and ½ of Cloves. Apply as a hot application (poultice) as directed above.

3. Use the herbs as indicated under LINIMENT.

SKIN LOTION

1. Soak 1 tbsp. each of finely cut Bloodroot, St. Johnswort flowers, and Marigold flowers in 8 oz. of 90% alcohol. Allow to stand for 10 days and stir occasionally. Strain through absorbent cotton and add 2 oz. Witch Hazel extract, 1 oz. glycerin and enough lime water to make 16 oz. (a pint). Shake well before using. (In the absence of Bloodroot, use the fall-collected bark or heavier stems of Sweet Fern.)

2. General hand lotion: (a) Prepare a jelly by gently simmering 2 tsp. of Irish Moss and one of Quince seeds in a pint of hot water for ½ hour and straining the cooled mixture. Add 1 oz. each glycerin and alcohol. Shake well before using. For winter use incorporate 2 tsp. of tincture benzoin compound, adding 10–15 drops at a time and each time shaking the bottle vigorously.

(b) Before preparing the jelly, the water content may be substituted with the following decoction. Simmer 2 tbsp. of Sweet Fern and Oak (both collected in late fall) in 1½ pts. of hot water until approximately ⅔ of the liquid (1 pint) remains. In the absence of either, one tsp. of pekoe tea may be substituted. Good for fresh burns, sunburn, skin irritations, etc.

(c) For a more astringent effect, include in above (b) formula ½ tbsp. of any two: Wild Geranium, Cinquefoil, Sumac bark, or Witch Hazel.

POISON IVY LOTION

Boil vigorously a large handful each of Sweet Fern twigs, Cinquefoil, Oak bark (or Wild Geranium) in a quart of hot water down to half quantity. Allow to cool and strain. Apply the solution as a wet compress every hour. Refrigerate.

This lotion is good for recent scratches and sores. Use it also as noted under the ASTRINGENT formula.

SKIN OINTMENT

1. Simmer for ½ hour 1 oz. each of Marsh Mallow (or Mallow) leaves or root and Elm bark in 2 oz. each of unsalted lard and beeswax, previously melted. Strain into a clean jar and stir until cold. Preserve in the refrigerator.

2. Simmer ½ hour 1 tbsp. each of Shepherd's Purse, Plantain leaves, and St. Johnswort flowers in a melted mixture containing 3 oz. unsalted lard (or mutton suet), 2 oz. beeswax, and 1 oz. of rosin. A few drops of tincture benzoin compound may also be added to each ounce of the strained, cold finished product. In the absence of either herb, Balm of Gilead buds may be used.

3. Simmer for a half-hour one heaping tbsp. of dried ground Plantain leaves and Shepherd's Purse in 4 ounces of unsalted lard or mutton suet. Strain through cheesecloth into ounce containers.

4. Plantain and gall ointment: Simmer 1 oz. of the powdered or finely ground Oak galls and 1 oz. of finely ground Plantain leaves (late fall-collected) in 4 oz. of lard. Strain. Allow to cool and, as it congeals, add 1½ tsp. of tincture benzoin compound and stir well.

5. Oak gall: Melt together 2 tsp. each of lanolin and yellow wax, then 3 oz. of petroleum jelly (or

Vaseline). Stir until congealed and incorporate 1 oz. of powdered galls. Do not strain.

6. Simmer for 15 minutes 1 oz. or a small handful each of dried St. Johnswort and Marigold flowers in 4 oz. of melted lard or in equal portions of lard and lanolin. Stir occasionally. Strain warm through wide gauze into an ointment jar. Incorporate 4 or 5 drops of oil of Eucalyptus as it congeals.

For skin irritations, scratches, sores, insect bites, etc.

7. (a) Tincture: Cover 1 tbsp. each of above herbs and Cinquefoil (or Septfoil) with 5 oz. alcohol. Allow to steep for a week. Shake the bottle daily. Strain.
(b) Oil: In 6 oz. of warmed vegetable oil gently simmer for 20 minutes 1 oz. each of St. Johnswort and Marigold flowers and of finely ground Bayberry bark or Gold Thread. Allow to cool and strain.

Use either liquid as indicated in #6.

8. Elder flower cream: Simmer for 1 hour 1 oz. Yellow Dock or Burdock root and 2 oz. Elder flowers in 2 oz. unsalted lard. Strain and incorporate 2 oz. cold cream. Excellent for acne, blackheads, pimples, etc.

If the skin problem (acne, psoriasis, etc.) is due to internal organic problems or malfunction, use one of the BLOOD PURIFIER remedies.

SLEEPING AID OR SEDATIVE

Mix equal parts of Scullcap, Lady's Slipper, Hops, Catnip, and Black Cohosh (optional). Mix a tsp. in a cup of hot water for 6–8 minutes and strain. Drink one cupful 2–3 hours before retiring and a second cupful one hour before. Also recommended is a brisk 20 minutes' walk an hour before bedtime, after drinking the herb tea.

SORE THROAT (QUINSY)

Use Self-Heal and Life Everlasting, a small handful of each simmered in a quart of hot water for 15–20 minutes. Use warm every hour. (See GARGLE and ASTRINGENT formulae.) Take internally for diarrhea, a tbsp. (tepid-cold) 3–4 times a day. This solution may also be used as an injection for hemorrhoids. Use equal parts of herbs noted under ASTRINGENT.

STOMACHIC

1. Mix 3 parts of Chamomile, 2 parts of Mint, and

½ each of Gentian and Gold Thread. Steep 1 tsp. in a cup of hot water. Drink cold a wineglassful ½ hour before and after meals.

2. Mix equal parts of Wild Cherry, Boneset, Mallow, Catnip, and Gentian, and ⅛ part of Quassia. Steep a tsp. in a cup of hot water until cool. Drink cold one strained cupful every 4–6 hours.

3. Mix equal parts of Boneset and Mallow or Hollyhock leaves and boil a cupful in a quart of hot water for 10 minutes. Remove from heat and add 2 tbsp. Mint and cut Angelica or Masterwort root. Cover until cool. Stir and strain. Take a tablespoonful every 3 or 4 hours with a little tepid water.

TISANE

This is a healthful substitute for pekoe tea, full of nutrients and minus the harmful, heart-stimulating caffeine. Use Alfalfa, Catnip, Chamomile, Red Clover, Sweet Clover, Elder flowers, Goldenrod, Linden, Pennyroyal, Peppermint and other Mints, Raspberry leaf, Rose leaf and fruit, Sassafras, Strawberry leaf, early summer Sweet Fern, Verbena, Wintergreen, and Yarrow. Use also the dried peels of lemon, orange, tangerine, and grapefruit and whatever of culinary herbs you like, such as Sage, Marjoram, Basil, Thyme. Mix equal portions of the herbs you prefer and steep a tsp. in a cup of hot water. Cover for 7–8 minutes. Stir and strain. *Sip slowly.*

TONER ("TONIC") OR GENERAL BODY CONDITIONER

1. "Spring Tonic": Boil 1 oz. each of Boneset, Burdock, Dandelion, and Sarsaparilla in a quart of hot water down to half. Drink cold a wineglassful 4 times a day.

2. See BLOOD PURIFIER #1.

3. Add Gentian and Gold Thread to either #1 or #2 above.

TOOTHACHE

See DENTAL POULTICE.

There is still another way of taking herbs. Once powdered, herbs provide measured doses which may be taken as often as their teas, via the druggist's empty gelatin capsules. The required herbs may be either powdered in a coffee or spice mill and sifted carefully through a sieve, flour sifter, or several folds of cheese cloth; or the powder may be obtained from an herbalist or herb dealer. (Add the remaining coarse stems and stubborn leaf portions to your everyday herb mixture.)

Note well the proportions of any given remedy. A formula calling for 3 parts (e.g. 3 ounces or 3 tablespoonsful) each of catnip, mint, fennel, and 1 each of boneset and yarrow requires that each ingredient—leaf, flower, or seed—is weighed separately and then all powdered parts are mixed together. *To avoid possible overdoses, do not initially measure each ingredient by its powder but by the original herb: the whole leaf, flower, or seed.* Since roots cannot be powdered in a spice mill, their powders must be obtained from commercial sources.

The mixture of powdered herbs is now ready for encapsulating. Obtain 100 empty gelatin #00 capsules from your pharmacist. Separate the capsule parts. Tap the larger part onto the powder until no more is taken up. Into the smaller part, insert only enough to fill the rounded end and then push together the two parts of the capsule until they fit snugly.

The average daily dose is that of the infusion: If taken three times a day, take one capsule three times a day with tepid water.

Bibliography

Ackerknecht, Erwin H. *A Short History of Medicine.* The Ronald Press, New York, 1955.

Arber, Agnes. *Herbals, Their Origins and Evolution,* 2nd edition. University Press, Cambridge, England, 1938.

Bardswell, Francis A. *The Herb Garden.* Adam and Charles Black, London, 1911.

Barnes, Henry Elmer. *Intellectual and Cultural History of the Western World.* The Cordon Co., New York, 1937.

Beach, Wooster. *The American Practice or The Family Physician.* New York, 1847.

Black, W. G. *Folk Medicine.* E. Stock, London, 1883.

Boas, Franz. *General Anthropology.* D. C. Heath & Co., New York, 1938.

Britton, N. Lord, and Addison Brown. *Illustrated Flora of the Northern United States and Canada,* 3 vols. Charles Scribner's Sons, New York, 1896.

Brown, O. Phelps. *The Compleat Herbalist.* Jersey City, New Jersey, 1865.

Burton, Robert. *Anatomy of Melancholy* (1621), ed. by Floyd Dell and Paul Jordan-Smith. Tudor Publishing Co., New York, 1932.

Candolle, Alphonse de. *Origin of Cultivated Plants* (2nd ed. 1886). Hafner Publishing Co., New York, 1964.

Carque, Otto. *Facts About Foods.* Natural Brands, Los Angeles, 1964.

Ciba Symposium (George E. Rosen, ed.), vol. 5, nos. 5 and 6 (1943). Ciba Pharmaceutical Products, Summit, New Jersey.

Clinical Excerpts, vol. 15, no. 3. Winthrop Chemical Co., New York, 1941.

Clute, William Nelson. *Plant Names*. E.P. Dutton & Co., New York, 1932.

Clymer, R. Swinburne. *Nature's Healing Agents*. Dorrance & Co., Philadelphia, 1963.

Coats, Alice M. *Flowers and Their History*. Pitman Publishing Corp., New York, 1956.

Coles, William. *The Art of Simpling*. London, 1657.

Croll, Oswald. *Basilica Chymica*. London, 1670.

Crops in Peace and War, Yearbook of Agriculture 1950–1951. United States Department of Agriculture.

Culpepper, Nicholas. *The English Physician*. London, 1826.

Dana, Mrs. William Starr. *How to Know the Wild Flowers*. Charles Scribner's Sons, New York, 1893.

Economic Botany, Journal of (1970). A publication of the Society of Economic Botany, published by The New York Botanical Garden at Lawrence, Kansas.

Ellacombe, Henry N. *Plant Lore and Garden Craft of Shakespeare*. Edward Arnold, London, 1896.

Emmart, Emily Walcott. *The Badianus Manuscript*. The Johns Hopkins Press, Baltimore, 1940.

Fenton, William N. *Contacts between Iroquois Herbalism and Colonial Medicine*. Smithsonian Institution, Washington, 1942.

Fielding, William J. *Strange Superstitions and Magical Practices*. The Blakiston Company, Philadelphia, 1945.

Frazer, Sir James George. *The Golden Bough*. The Macmillan Co., New York, 1942.

Garrison, Fielding H. *Introduction to a History of Medicine*. W. B. Saunders, Philadelphia, 1925.

Georgia, Ada E. *A Manual of Weeds*. Macmillan Co., New York, 1925.

Gerard, John. *The Herball or General Historie of Plants*. London, 1597.

Gilmore, Melvin. *Indian Lore*. Ithaca, New York, 1930.

Gordon, Benjamin Lee. *Medicine Throughout Antiquity*. F.A. Davis Co., Philadelphia, 1949.

————. *The Romance of Medicine*. F.A. Davis Co., Philadelphia, 1949.

Greene, Thomas. *Universal Herbal,* 2 vols. London, 1823.

Grieve, M. *A Modern Herbal,* 2 vols. Harcourt, Brace & Co., New York, 1931.

Guillet, Alma C. *Make Friends of Trees and Shrubs*. Doubleday and Co., Garden City, 1962.

Haggard, H. W. *The Doctor in History*. Yale University Press, New Haven, 1934.

———. *Devils, Drugs and Doctors.* Harper and Row, New York, 1945.

Harper, S. F. *Prescriber and Clinical Repertory of Medicinal Herbs.* Homeopathic Publishing Co., London, 1938.

Harris, Ben Charles. *Better Health with Culinary Herbs,* Barre Publishers, Barre, Mass., 1971.

———. *Eat the Weeds,* Barre Publishers, 1969.

———. *Kitchen Medicines,* Barre Publishers, 1968.

Health from Herbs (T. Bartram, ed.), April and June 1956. Leicester, England.

Hertzler, Joyce Oramel. *The History of Utopian Thought.* The Macmillan Co., New York, 1923.

Hogstad, Anton Jr. *Drugs of the North American Indian.* Merck & Co., Rahway, New Jersey, (no date).

———. *The Romance of Drugs.* Merck & Co. (no date).

Hunter, John D. *Manners and Customs of Several Indian Tribes.* J. Maxwell Co., Philadelphia, 1823.

Hylander, Clarence J. *The World of Plant Life.* The Macmillan Co., New York, 1939.

Inglis, Brian. *A History of Medicine.* World Publishing Co., New York, 1965.

Journal of Natural Products, vol. 33, nos. 1, 2, 3, 4. The American Society of Pharmacognosy and The Lloyd Library and Museum, Cincinnati.

Karel, Leonard, and Elizabeth Spencer Roach. *A Dictionary of Antibiosis.* Columbia University Press, New York, 1951.

Lang, W. H., ed. *A Text-Book of Botany.* The Macmillan Company, New York, 1903.

LaWall, Charles H. *4000 Years of Pharmacy.* Lippincott Publishing Co., Philadelphia, 1927.

Leyel, C. F. *Cinquefoil,* Faber and Faber, London, 1951.

———. *The Elixirs of Life,* Faber and Faber, London, 1948.

———. *The Magic of Herbs,* Harcourt, Brace & Co., New York, 1926.

Ligeros, K. A. *How Ancient Healing Governs Modern Therapeutics.* G.P. Putnam & Sons, New York, 1937.

Lindley, John. *Flora Medica,* London, 1938.

Lloyd Library, Bulletin of, no. 4, Pharmacy Series. Cincinnati, 1911.

Lounsberry, Alice. *A Guide to the Trees.* Frederick A. Stokes Co., New York, 1900.

Maddox, John Lee. *The Medicine Man.* The Macmillan Company, New York, 1923.

Mason, Otis T. *Origins of Inventions*. London, 1901.

The Medical Herbalist, (J.R. Yemm, ed.), vol. XI, August 1935–July 1937. National Association of Medical Herbalists of Great Britain.

Meyer, J. E. *The Herbalist and Herb Doctor*. Indiana Botanic Gardens, Hammond, Indiana, 1934.

Meyrick, William. *The New Family Herbal*. London, 1740.

Moldenke, Harold N. and Alma L. *Plants of the Bible*. The Ronald Press Company, New York, 1952.

Mooney, James, and Frank M. Olbrechts. *The Swimmer Manuscript*, Bulletin 99. Bureau of American Ethnology, Smithsonian Institute, Washington, 1932.

Muenscher, Walter C. *Weeds*. The Macmillan Company, New York, 1935.

Osler, Sir William. *The Evolution of Modern Medicine*. Yale University Press, New Haven, 1921.

Payne, Joseph Frank. *English Medicine in Anglo-Saxon Times*. The Clarendon Press, Oxford, England, 1904.

Peterson, Maude Gridley. *How to Know Wild Fruits*. The Macmillan Co., New York, 1905.

The Pharmaceutical Recipe Book, 3rd edition. American Pharmaceutical Association, 1943.

Philbrick, Helen, and Richard Gregg. *Companion Plants and How to Use Them*. Devin-Adair Co., New York, 1966.

Podolsky, Edward. *Medicine Marches On*. Harper Bros., New York, 1934.

Pomet, Pierre. *History of Drugs*. London, 1748.

Porta, Giovanni Battista della. *Natural Magick* (1658). Basic Books, Inc., New York, 1957.

Price, Weston. *Nutrition and Physical Degeneration*. P.B. Hoeber, Inc., New York, 1939.

Prior, R. C. A. *Popular Names of British Plants*. Frederic Norgate, London, 1879.

Quinn, Vernon. *Leaves, Their Place in Life and Legend*. Frederick Stokes Co., New York, 1937.

Reed, Howard S. *A Short History of the Plant Sciences*. Chronica Botanica Co., Waltham, Mass., 1942.

Ritzenthaler, Robert E. *The Oneida Indians of Wisconsin*, vol. 19, no. 1. Museum of the City of Milwaukee, 1950.

Robinson, Victor. *The Story of Medicine*. A. and C. Boni Co.. New York, 1931.

Rohde, Eleanor Sinclair. *A Garden of Herbs*. Hale, Cushman and Flint, Boston, 1936.

Bibliography

Saunders, Charles F. *Useful Wild Plants of the United States and Canada*. Robert M. McBride Co., New York, 1920.

Scully, Virginia. *A Treasury of American Indian Herbs*. Crown Publishers, Inc., New York, 1970.

Shryock, Richard H. *Development of Modern Medicine*. University of Pennsylvania, Philadelphia, 1936.

———. *Medicine in America*. Johns Hopkins Press, Baltimore, 1966.

Sigerist, Henry E. *The Great Doctors*. W. W. Norton Co., New York, 1933.

———. *A History of Medicine*. Oxford University Press, New York, 1951.

Skinner, Charles M. *Myths and Legends of Flowers, Trees, Fruits and Plants*. J.B. Lippincott, Philadelphia, 1911.

Smith, A. W. *A Gardener's Book of Plant Names*. Harper and Row, New York, 1963.

Smith, Huron B. *Ethnobotany of the Ojibwe Indians*. Bulletin of the Public Museum of the City of Milwaukee, 1932.

Spencer, Edwin Rollin. *Just Weeds*. Charles Scribner's Sons, New York, 1940.

Stedman, Thomas Lathrop. *Medical Dictionary*. William Woods Co., Baltimore, 1934.

Swanton, John R. *Indian Tribes of the Lower Mississippi Valley*, Bulletin 43, U.S. Bureau of American Ethnology, Washington.

———. *Source Material for the Social and Ceremonial Life of the Choctaw Indians*, Bulletin 103, U.S. Bureau of American Ethnology, Washington, 1931.

Thiselton-Dyer, T. F. *The Folklore of Plants*. Chatto & Windus, London, 1889.

Thompson, J. M. *New Testament Miracles*. E. Arnold, London, 1912.

Thorndyke, Lynn. *A History of Magic and Experimental Science*, vols. 5, 6, 7, 8. Columbia University Press, New York, 1958.

Thornwald, Jurgen. *Science and Secrets of Early Medicine*. Harcourt, Brace and World, Inc., New York, 1962.

Turner, William. *The Newe Herball*. London, 1562.

Vogel, Virgil J. *American Indian Medicine*. University of Oklahoma Press, Norman, Oklahoma, 1970.

Waddle, C. W. "Miracles of Healing," *American Journal of Psychology*, vol. 20, April 1909.

Walsh, James J. *Old-Time Makers of Medicine*. Fordham University Press, New York, 1911.

White, Ellen G. *Counsels on Diet and Foods*. Review and Herald Publishing Association, Takoma Park, Washington, D.C., 1938.

Wood, Horatio C., and Arthur Osol. *The Dispensatory of the United States of America*. J.B. Lippincott Co., Philadelphia, 1943.

Woodville, William. *Medical Botany,* 2nd edition, vol. 1. London, 1810.

Youngken, Heber W. *Pharmaceutical Botany,* 6th edition. P. Blakiston's Sons & Co., Philadelphia, 1938.

———. *Textbook of Pharmacognosy,* 6th edition. The Blakiston Co., Philadelphia, 1948.

Glossary

ADJUVANT That which is added to a remedy to assist or increase the action of the main ingredient.

ALTERATIVE Helps to alter or gradually correct the symptoms of minor functional disorders of the system. Also called "blood purifier."

AMENORRHEA Absence or suppression of the menses, from causes other than pregnancy or menopause.

ANALGESIC Helps to relieve pain.

ANEMIA A condition in which the blood is reduced in amount or is deficient in red blood-cells or in hemoglobin.

ANODYNE Helps to quiet or relieve pain.

ANTHELMINTIC An agent which expels or kills intestinal worms.

ANTIBIOTIC Helps to destroy pathogenic action of microbes.

ANTICATARRHAL Prevents the formation of or aids in the removal of catarrh, prevents the inflammation of the mucous membranes.

ANTICOLIC Prevents or reduces colic, helps to prevent spasmodic pains in the stomach.

ANTIDYSPEPTIC Improves or prevents poor digestion.

ANTILITHIC Prevents the formation of stone (gravel) in the kidney apparatus.

ANTIPERIODIC Reduces feverish conditions and prevents the recurrence of similar symptoms.

ANTIRHEUMATIC An agent useful in rheumatism, lumbago, arthritis, or gout, or in the prevention or healing of such a condition.

ANTISCORBUTIC Used in the prevention or treatment of scurvy.

ANTISPASMODIC Allays or helps to prevent the recurrence of spasms, temporarily relieving muscular irritability and excessive contraction.

AROMATIC Possesses an agreeable and fragrant odor, plus mildly stimulative properties.

ARTHRITIS Inflammation of a joint.

ASTRINGENT Has the property of coagulating blood and drawing together or binding the tissues, thus checking discharges. Today many astringents are valued for their antibiotic principles. (*See* VULNERARY.)

BILIOUSNESS An ailment caused or evidenced by trouble with the bile or liver, resulting in digestive disturbance.

BITTER(S) A mild stomachic tonic used to improve digestion.

BLOOD PURIFIER *See* ALTERATIVE.

BRONCHITIS Inflammation of the mucous membrane of the bronchial system.

CANKER An ulcerous sore, or minute vesicles on the tongue, cheek, or lips.

CARMINATIVE Expels gas from bowels, stomach, and intestines; helps to overcome colic and flatulence and to prevent griping.

CATARRH Simple inflammation of a mucous membrane, especially of the respiratory tract.

CATHARTIC A vigorous laxative used in constipation. Not recommended since it may tend to irritate the system. (*See* LAXATIVE.)

CHOLESTEROL A fat-like substance found in bile and gallstones and deposited by the excessive ingestion of fatty meats, egg yolks, and other protein foods.

COLIC A cramp or spasmodic pain in the stomach or intestines.

CYSTITIS Inflammation of the urinary bladder.

DECOCTION The process of boiling herbs in order to extract their principles; the resulting liquid.

DEMULCENT Allays the action of stimulating or acrid substances and overactive herbs, and is soothing to the irritated mucous membranes. Thus, desirable in ordinary colds, coughs, and diarrhea, and as a required ingredient of laxative and diuretic herb mixtures.

DEOBSTRUENT Removes obstructions from the various organs.

DEPURATIVE Removes waste products from the body.

DIAPHORETIC Increases the perspiration; an aid in eliminating waste products through the skin. Should be taken in moderate doses and only until the desired result has been obtained. Diaphoretics taken profusely may tend to exhaust the user.

DIGESTANT An aid in the digestion of food.

DIURETIC Helps to increase the flow of urine and to improve or increase elimination of the waste products of the body through the urine.

DROPSY An excessive and unnatural accumulation of watery fluid in any subcutaneous tissues or cavity of the body.

DYSMENORRHEA Painful and difficult menstruation.

DYSPEPSIA Indigestion; impaired digestion, accompanied by nausea, heartburn, and acrid belching.

ECZEMA An inflammatory disorder of the skin presenting multiform lesions, moist or dry, and often accompanied with itching and burning sensation.

EMETIC Causes vomiting.

EMOLLIENT Used externally to exert a healing or soothing effect on the skin.

EXPECTORANT Helps to facilitate the expulsion of mucus from the respiratory tract.

FEBRIFUGE Helps to check or expel fever.

FLATULENCE The state of being affected with the presence of excessive gas in the alimentary canal.

GASTRITIS Inflammation of the stomach's mucous lining.

GLUTINOUS Having the quality of glue; viscous, sticky.

GRAVEL The formation in the urinary passages of very small concretions or calculi.

HEPATIC An aid in liver disorders.

INFUSION The process of steeping herbs in hot water in order to extract its soluble principles; the herb tea obtained by this process.

JAUNDICE A pathological condition characterized by a yellowish staining of the blood, the skin, the whites of the eyes, the deeper tissues, and the secretions with bile pigments.

LAXATIVE Helps to correct constipation by moderately increasing bowel action.

LEUCORRHEA A whitish, viscid discharge from the vagina, resulting from the inflammation or irritation of that organ.

MUCILAGINOUS Gummy or sticky, usually soothing to inflamed areas.

NEPHRITIS Inflammation of the kidneys.

NERVINE Affects the nervous system and tends to quiet a temporary nervous irritation due to excitement, fatigue, overstrain, or headache.

PARTURIENT Relating to or being in the process of childbirth.

PLEURISY An inflammation of the membranes that envelop the thorax and lungs.

POULTICE Crushed or ground herbs moistened with hot water or vinegar, externally applied to an affected area.

PULMONARY Pertaining to or affecting the lungs.

PURGATIVE More drastic in action than a cathartic and therefore *not recommended*.

QUINSY   An inflammation of the throat or tonsils, attended by the formation of pus.

REFRIGERANT   Has a cooling and refreshing effect upon the system.

RELAXANT   An agent which relieves strain or tension.

RHEUMATISM   A painful inflammation and swelling of the muscles and joints.

SCROFULA   A constitutional disorder of a tubercular nature, causing a swelling of the lymph glands, especially of the neck, and inflaming the joints.

SEDATIVE   Allays nervous irritability and excitement, and exerts a soothing and quieting influence upon the nervous system, but has no narcotic effect. (*See* ANTISPASMODIC and NERVINE.)

SPASM   A sudden and involuntary contraction of a muscle or muscle fiber.

STIMULANT   Helps to increase the various functional actions of the body. Do not confuse this category with the harmful artificial stimulants such as tea, coffee, liquor, spices, smoking, etc.

STOMACHIC   Promotes appetite, stimulates gastric secretion and digestion, and strengthens and gives tone to the stomach. (*See* BITTER TONIC.)

SUDORIFIC   A strong diaphoretic intended to produce profuse perspiration. *Not recommended* because of its weakening effect upon the body.

TISANE   An infusion, an herb tea.

TONIC   Helps to restore tone to muscle tissue, being invigorating and strengthening.

TONIC, BITTER   A popular or non-technical term for a digestive adjuvant; helps to improve or restore appetite and to increase the flow of the gastric juices.

UTERINE   Relating to the uterus, the womb.

VERMICIDE   An agent which kills intestinal parasitic worms.

VERMIFUGE   An agent which expels parasitic worms from the intestines.

VULNERARY   An agent useful in healing of wounds.

Index

Index 235

The Best Books on Health
LARCHMONT BOOKS

All You Should Know about Arthritis by Ruth Adams and Frank Murray. *What Adams and Murray have to say about arthritis.* 256 pages, $3.25.

Almonds to Zoybeans by "Mothey" Parsons. *The A to Z cookbook of quality protein meals without meat.* 192 pages, $1.50.

Beverages by Adams and Murray. *The advantages of choosing healthful beverages are the focus of this interesting book.* 288 pages, $1.75.

Body, Mind and the B Vitamins by Adams and Murray. *The most informative book ever written about the B vitamins and their essential role in mental and physical health.* 320 pages, $3.25.

The Compleat Herbal by Ben Charles Harris. *An authentic, comprehensive guide to medicinal plants and herbs.* 248 pages, $3.95.

The Complete Home Guide to All the Vitamins by Ruth Adams. *This popular and valuable home reference answers all your questions about vitamins.* 432 pages, $3.95.

Eating in Eden by Ruth Adams. *Learn to appreciate the joys and benefits of natural foods.* 206 pages, $1.75.

Fighting Depression by Harvey Ross, M.D. *This book contains valuable material for anyone suffering from depression.* 224 pages, $3.95.

Food for Beauty by Helena Rubenstein. *Frank Murray has revised and updated Miss Rubenstein's 1938 classic on diet and beauty.* 256 pages, $1.95.

The Good Seeds, the Rich Grains, the Hardy Nuts for a Happier, Healthier Life by Adams and Murray. *This book cracks all the myths about the value of over-processed foods.* 352 pages, $1.75.

Health Foods by Adams and Murray. *This complete mini-encyclopedia tells all about health foods.* 352 pages, $3.95.

How to Control Your Allergies by Robert Forman, Ph.D. *Helps you find out which chemical or natural allergen is causing discomfort and how to live healthfully with an allergy.* 256 pages, $3.95.

Is Low Blood Sugar Making You a Nutritional Cripple? by Adams and Murray. *The latest information about hypoglycemia, including the proper diet and supplements.* 176 pages, $3.50.

Lose Weight, Feel Great! by John Yudkin, M.D., Ph.D. *This book describes the healthful diet for those who want to lose pounds and inches permanently. 220 pages. $1.75.*

Megavitamin Therapy by Adams and Murray. *Describes this great breakthrough in treatment for alcoholics, schizophrenics, drug addicts, and hyperactive children. 286 pages, $3.25.*

Minerals: Kill or Cure? by Adams and Murray. *The first complete book ever written about minerals and their essential place in a healthful diet. 368 pages, $1.95.*

The New High Fiber Diet by Adams and Murray. *This book contains important information on the value of fiber in your diet and includes over 250 delicious high fiber recipes. 320 pages, $2.25.*

Program Your Heart for Health by Frank Murray. *One of the most current books on the role of proper nutrition in preventing heart attack or stroke. Valuable information on a vital subject. 368 pages, $2.95.*

Vitamin B12 and Folic Acid by Adams and Murray. *Learn why these two B vitamins are so necessary to good health. 160 pages, $1.95.*

The Vitamin B6 Book by Adams and Murray. *Detailed information on the many benefits pyridoxine provides: prevention of strokes, convulsions, anemia, protection against ill effects of The Pill. 160 pages, $1.75.*

The Larchmont
PREVENTIVE HEALTH LIBRARY

The **Preventive Health Library** has been designed to give you all the facts concerning the uses and effects of a particular supplement in a handy, easy-to-read format that is highlighted to help you digest key concepts, All books are by Adams and Murray, the famous health team who keep you informed on the most valuable health topics.

Improving Your Health with Vitamin A. 128 pages, $1.25.

Improving Your Health with Vitamin C. 160 pages, $1.50.

Improving Your Health with Calcium and Phosphorus. 128 pages, $1.25.

Improving Your Health with Vitamin E. 176 pages, $1.50.

Improving Your Health with Niacin (Vitamin B₃). 128 pages, $1.75.

Improving Your Health with Zinc. 128 pages, $1.50.

LARCHMONT BOOKS
6255 Barfield Rd.
Atlanta, Ga. 30328